Enjoy Vity

Also by J.Yves Verheyen

Healing water

J.Yves Verheyen

EnjoyVity, your full spectrum of life

This book is designed to provide accurate and authoritative information about personal well being. Neither the author nor the publisher is engaged in rendering medical, legal, or other professional services by publishing this book. If any such assistance is required, the services of a qualified medical or other professional should be sought. The author and publisher will not be responsible for any liability, loss, or risk incurred as a result of the use and application of any of the information contained in this book. While the author has made every effort to provide accurate references and Internet addresses at the time of publication, neither the publisher nor the author assumes any responsibility for errors or for changes that occur after publication.

Links to persons and organizations found at this site are provided solely as a service to our users. These links do not constitute an endorsement of these persons or organizations or their programs by the author and none should be inferred. The author is not responsible for the content of the individual organization Web pages found at these links.

Copyright © 2010 by J.Yves Verheyen All Rights Reserved
ISBN: 978-2-9601022-0-8
Published in Europe by Verheyen Consulting.
www.enjoyvity.com

Never disregard professional medical advice or delay in seeking it because of something you have read in this book.

The information does not intentionally mention brand names, nor does it endorse any particular products.

Foreword

Everyone is born a genius, but the process of living de-geniuses them.
~ R. Buckminster Fuller

Yes we have a meaningful contribution to make. Show there is hope for the generations to come, that we can team up for a better world, a better me and a better you. We want you to become re-optimistic.

> "We are part of a positive minded team
>
> We question ourselves since decennia, centuries, millennia
>
> We search for the truth
>
> Whatever deep water we get in
>
> We will stay cool and understand we need to help others
>
> Changes are of all times
>
> There is no way back
>
> We don't look for an escape as we are 'the bridge'
>
> To a new era
>
> We owe this to mankind
>
> To ourselves
>
> That is why we are around"

EnjoyVity is intended for those who want to enhance their life and safeguard that of their beloved ones. So whatever age you are at now you can seriously benefit from the many subjects laid out in this book. For sure you will benefit much more the younger you are, but only when implementing some or the mayor part of the given knowledge.

Also for those 100 million and ever growing number of men and women, wherever they may live, who adapted the modern western way of living and eating and will be or are interested to be over 85 and healthy in just some decades from now.

For the over 220 million Baby Boomers (1945-1960) in the United States, Canada, Europe, Australia and New Zealand (of which 78 million* in US alone), the 46million (US alone) Generation-X (1965-1980) and the 70 million (US alone) Generation-Y (1981-1990).

*The Alzheimer's Association® estimates that 10 million Boomers in the United States and over 15 million in Europe will develop Alzheimer's disease. We don't want that to happen to all of you.

We are not talking about cheap 3 minute solutions, but if you INVEST now 5 hours of your precious time we show you how to gain step by step many 1000 minutes and many more $/€ (*).

(*)Expenditures in the United States on health care surpassed $2 trillion in 2006, over eight times the $253 billion spent in 1980. In 2006, U.S. health care spending was about $7,026 per resident and accounted for 16% of the nation's Gross Domestic Product (GDP). We will not only help the State (which is partly you, right) to save greatly on this exploding budget, but more important show you how to avoid personally the health care services and its growing costs to you.

How much do you spend on food, drinks, your look, your health, commuting ... - not to mention the countless hours you spend in front of TV or in your bed? Yes, you were right to invest now some hours to improve your mental and physical health and to shape your healthy future and **assure your youthful aging!**

Dedicated to You
MAY THIS BOOK BRING YOU SOME IMPORTANT MISSING PIECES TO THE PUZZLE OF YOUR LIFE!

Note this is not about a DIET, not Science-Fiction, not a Novel.

1. Introduction

> Its all about remembering
> Where did you come from
> You were, are and will be spirit
> You are never alone   ~unknown

Of course it has all been thought off, said, invented, written and also forgotten, probably even more than once, before. Collective memory loss or amnesia is of all times. Let's remember!

It is also partly about de-fragmentation of existing but scattered information and knowledge, about re-building and re-formatting the puzzle of life.

It is about invisible trees in the forest. Meaning too many research studies, figures lead to different conclusions leading to confusion, an insolvable puzzle and even immobilization.

And about your spirit, motivation at the moment you were trying to assimilate or practice some related information. Maybe you were not ready for your new road.

In case you knew already and agree upon, which is not our first goal, all that we serve you within this work, you will still enjoy the ride as it will refresh your mind, keep you focused and make you part of a team which is enjoying all challenges of life. Research has proven that having a strong network of friends, family and community is key to longevity. If certain advices seem too obvious then still question yourself if you already integrated them in your life. Who doesn't need reminders anyway.

Even in case you tried it all before and became desperate and suspicious the reading will comfort you and get you in a fresh state of mind and will build your self-confidence, knowing that there is always a way out.

So grab this dynamic cocktail for your life's enhancement as a summary 'again'. Read it at your wish chapter by chapter or in random order, after all it is your decision, your book and more important your unique life.

Within "EnjoyVity" you will find the 7 steps which will guide you towards a healthy and successful long life. At the end of each chapter you will find a 'remember' quote and a summarized advice on possible added life-years.

First de-stress and get prepared for better reading and remembering: find a quiet moment and place, close your eyes, focus on your belly breathing, relax your lower jaw, touch with the tongue point the upper palate behind the front teeth, breath slowly in through your nose towards your stomach (diaphragm), keep your breath half that time while (firmly) pressing your tongue now at the indicated spot on your upper palate and exhale slowly through your mouth while using your abdominal muscles to push the air and toxins out. **Yawning** allowed and if exercise is done correctly it will definitely be part of it. Repeat 6 to 8 times. More *on the subject under chapter 13.*

Now! I want you to start from the back. Read first the back-flap and then the content of this book (page 219). Only then decide which chapter inspires you most and start there.

At the start of your day, drive, lesson, ... and also at the start of your reading spend a few minutes on the special 'zero-neck-roll' movements as described in chapter 4 to improve your vision and awareness.

We suggest you read a chapter a day and finish the book within 20 to 30 days, then practice whatever you found of interest in it for another 30 days and then preferably report/comment/testify on our website www.enjoyvity.com

This scenario of 'de-stress/back-flap/content' ('DBC') will work best for any reading or other learning process. You will gain great time and probably also money as you will increase conscious, understand and assimilate faster and remember the information much longer.

Discover the missing piece in your puzzle...

Get to it with Mark Twain:

> "Twenty years from now you will be more disappointed
> by the things that you didn't do than by the ones you did do.
> So throw off the bowlines. Sail away from the safe harbor.
> Catch the trade winds in your sails.
> **Explore. Dream. Discover.**"

Lets only add: **"Enjoy"!**

Indeed stand, sit or lie back and enjoy the reading, the journey.

This not about a diet, it is not a novel or science fiction.
You can even read this as a fairy tale. Go back to your ancestor roots, find your

base.
What did I come to do here?
What is my task? My motto?
What is there prepared for me?

Start dreaming ...positive change is coming.

It is faith and destiny which brought you here, follow your intuition

You made the right decision.

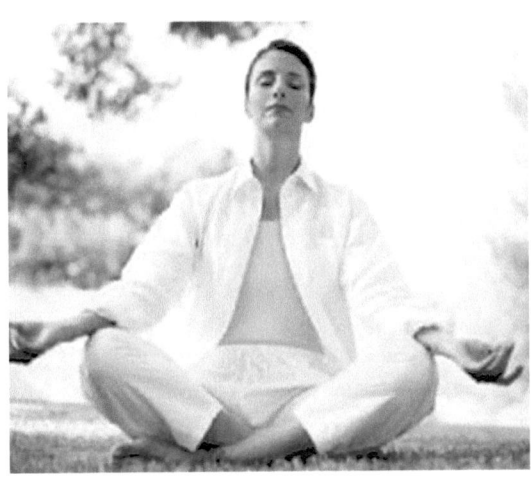

2. Live and make Your life

Progress is impossible without change, and those who cannot change their minds, cannot change anything.   ~ George Bernard Shaw

Correct! Make 'your' life, not that of others! Nobody, except for your close family, maybe, will build your life and future without direct self-profit, why would you then concentrate on creating that of others. Go around or dump 'people consumers'. Make your life a balanced giving-receiving experience. Be in the driver's seat, or better make it a comfortable coach.

Know where you stand economically, financially, socially, physically, spiritually, emotionally, ...

Understand Robert Kiyosaki's message in 'Rich dad, Poor dad' where he states that the poor and middle class work for money, either as employee or self-employed independent, but the rich as business owners or investors have money work for them to heart. Thus financial freedom is not waiting at the end of the corporate ladder. Step out of the crowd; get informed at 'richdad.com' , a must these days.

Explore!

Life is, like you prefer, as a cold torrent or a choky tropical waterfall, it gurgles or thunders alongside, always too fast, but fascinating, grandiose, powerful and unforgettable for conscious lovers.

Don't live just to work! The majority of the people are raised, educated, trained, obliged and even forced to concentrate on their work. Even with an actually limited and contested 36 hours working week the 'commute-work-sleep'- or 'metro-boulo(t)-dodo'-timing, as the French say, fills up for most 5 days out of 7. The remaining time is needed for recuperating, meaning watch TV, consuming and overspending (as intentionally programmed by the divine super-capitalism marketing) the gained income.

There is a road out towards a sustainable and equitable world. Just look around, get informed, be and act consciously. Let's get involved. For a starter watch the learning and funny video's at 'storyofstuff.com'.

Define and adjust when needed your true spending needs and life goals. There is no specific road without a defined destination. Step out of the crowd. A better life with less but more enriching work should be the target! Without although losing your commitment.

Don't be an average person. All official figures about income and even life expectancy are average figures and the difference between the lows and highs are important. Strive towards the upper end. We want to add vigor to your entire extended life. The **"EnjoyVity"** approach wants boost life expectancy, with 5, 10 or more years, of individuals, but also of the population in general. We want to show that the 4th age can be bright, fun and that enjoying the 5th will be at reach for many soon.

Know or define what internal feelings you are really after.
Is it fulfillment, well-being, connection, love, peace, ..., or joy.

Find your flame.

Find first out if you are a morning or evening type. Morning people wake up early and are most alert in the first part of the day, and evening people are most alert in the evening hours and prefer to go to bed late. Then choose your working time and hours consequently. Don't force your brain and body endlessly against this biological flow. Find ways to avoid rush hours and the common commuting paths. Move parallel, opposite or outside the known home-work-home stream as the latter became very time and energy consuming. Work from home or within your neighborhood whenever possible. Strive towards making your life one long enriching vacation. Thus start being an intelligent and maximum 50% workaholic.

Invest in yourself first and continuously! Education does not stop while finishing (high-) school. Be an ongoing auto-didactic. Become your own private journalist and find your own truth and opinion.

Do not be satisfied with an 'I heard about it' or 'I looked at it' or 'I somewhat touched it' or 'I once tried it'. We will show and help you how to integrate positive thoughts and actions in your everyday life.

The days of a guaranteed lifetime carrier in a sole company are well over for most of us. Be flexible thus and start new projects over and over. Flexibility is the key to your overall wellbeing. Keep your body and mind in a receptive positive state. Understand that your life-road is well graven in your hand palm and not in a whatsoever temporary work-contract.

Question yourself! Are you walking through life with a smile? Are you happy? Are you satisfied? Are you complaining? Are you getting home tired after work? Are you jealous? Are you just surviving? Are you stressed? Are you exhausted while waking up? Are you seriously in debt? Are you sick? Are you burned out? Are you bored out?

Know yourself! Look in your 3-dimensional mirrors. How are friends, people, and colleagues defining you? Is that how you want to be seen? Is that really you? Is that how you see yourself? Are you comfortable in your skin? Listen to yourself. Listen to your heart. Listen to your inner you.

"Face your deficiencies and acknowledge them;
but do not let them master you.
Let them teach you patience, sweetness, insight."   ~Helen Keller

Be yourself! Be open to and for change. Having a positive attitude and creating positive daily habits will bring you closer to your objectives.
Have your 'plan B', always at hand in your personal drawer. Make a list of all positive and negative features that your actual occupation and/or life are holding.
Is there a balance or are the negative ones in majority? Find and write down 2 or 3 alternative approaches with their pros and cons.
Be inventive. Evaluate and act consequently.
If needed go back and resource or find finally your roots, origins and healthy future.

Never give up: "It won't matter that 10,000 doors might be slammed in your face, ..., because when door number 10,001 flies open, revealing pathways of jade and gardens of love, with flowers dancing, fountains sparkling, friends blushing, moonbeams beaming, and abundance abounding, you'll completely forget about all the other doors. Happens every day, The Universe", from 'tut.com'.

Likewise you should understand that there is always a new path which leads you to a never expected bright future. There are no limits to your wellbeing if only you are open-minded and believe in it. The truth is inside you. The universe is not pre-minded.

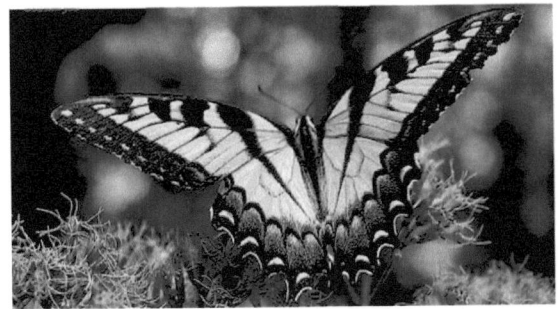

"To be in HARMONY is feeling
like a BUTTERFLY
on a sunny morning in May"

Grab your 'golden' life with both hands. Don't lose precious time by complaining or being negative.

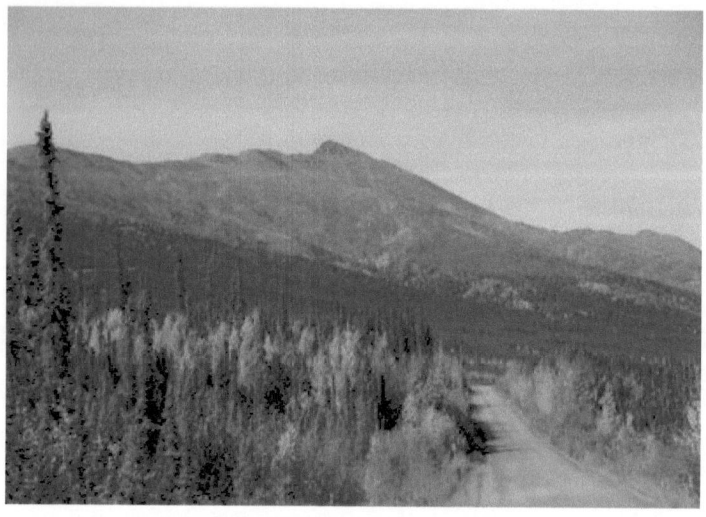

Find your path to paradise

Life should be and is 'easy'. The most difficult life questions can still be answered in a split second with a yes or no, which they will be, but by others for you if you remain undecided.
'Easy' means not without thoughts, as you have a dream, a target and a plan to reach them. So use your time consequently. Define and then concentrate on your 'productive' time which brings you income or the rewards you were expecting. The golden time who materializes your dreams and brings you wealth and wellness!

What is your goal in life? Write it down!
....
....
....

Scan and print it out, look at it and read it loud daily the first weeks.

"First, have a definite, clear practical ideal; a goal, an objective.
Second, have the necessary means to achieve your ends;
wisdom, money, materials, and methods.
Third, adjust all your means to that end." ~Aristoteles

Start with Your **Gold-Time-Management**.

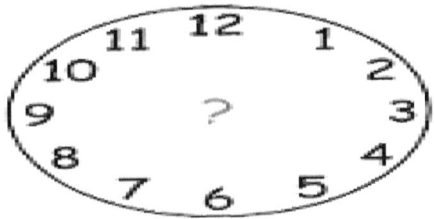

If you feel a need to **stretch your available time**, feel absorbed or used by time, ... or are just focused on your project, then learn to say NO.
You still can show others your concerns, empathy and remain positive. Remember that your time is your own. Don't let other people take control of your time. Minimize communication outside of the narrow (time) frame needed to fulfill both of your objectives.

If you have a hard time doing so then learn it while using your mirror, put a smile on your face and say: **'No, thank you!'**
Repeat 10 times loudly, you can shout or sing it: 'No, thank you!'

This not a negative approach, you and you only decide what to do in your 24 hours. So it is positive for yourself to think and say whenever you decide so:

"No, thank you I don't want to use my time on it."
Ok, you might have gained already an hour a day or a year or two in your lifetime, when using these 3 simple, clean words during your next conversation while having 'Your' future on focus.

Not bad, right? When you know that ... you should think that every hour of your time is worth minimum 1000 $/€/£/... Indeed a 1000 of your 'fill in your preferred' expensive currency (E.C.).

Why not? As a 50% workaholic you are going to work 20 hours/week and 10 months a year making you before cost and tax a sincere 800.000 of your E.C.! A minimum, as we said correctly.
So your first or next 'No, thank you!' will come with great decision, we are sure.
Also every hour you save commuting, administrating and organizing will get your mind and hands free to concentrate on your gold 'productive' time. You will keep on track towards your target and will have a clear blue sea of leisure time.

So from now on don't worry, stick to your life's target and follow your master-plan.

> **Be happy**! As happiness is the first and probably the only feeling you should aim for.

Living longer and healthier will then be a result instead of an unreachable goal. That is what "**EnjoyVity**" is about.

**We in the post-industrialized world made, in just a generation, exceptions the rule and common rules and behaviors became thus exceptions
~J. Yves Verheyen**

Some of those new rules are overconsumption, overeating, individual-ism, sedentary-ism, immobile-ism, unreal-ism, incivility-ism and ignore-ism.

The 4th world is mainly rural, agricultural and nomadic (www.cwis.org)
in the US only 21% is still rural
1.2 billion of the world's people live on less than what a dollar a day can buy
51% of world population lives in cities growing to 60% by 2030

Actual **top 10** of cities:
1. Tokyo, Japan - 28,025,000
2. Mexico City, Mexico - 18,131,000
3. Mumbai, India - 18,042,000
4. Sáo Paulo, Brazil - 17, 711,000
5. New York City, USA - 16,626,000
6. Shanghai, China - 14,173,000
7. Lagos, Nigeria - 13,488,000
8. Los Angeles, USA - 13,129,000
9. Calcutta, India - 12,900,000
10. Buenos Aires, Argentina - 12,431,000

To face the problems of runaway growth of cities in developing countries we need to find ways to stop the further drain to the city and invest in urban agriculture. Formerly all citizens had their small garden in the suburbs where they got their fresh food, relaxation and social network.

Your great puzzle of life might be acting around or in one of the above mentioned cities if we can show you where your missing piece is hidden within these pages we both will feel great and healthy.

Dare to change.
Dare to move.
Dare to be YOU.
Overcome the chaos involved with it.

Use Émile Coué de Châtaigneraie's autosuggestion:
"**Every day, in every way, I'm getting better and better**"

So remember say "No, thank you"
                to 'Metro-boulo-dodo'

        to negativity

So remember you can add years to your life

              by just saying "No, thank you"

              by feeling "Happy"

Note: All the links to websites with extra information about certain subjects are optional, use them at your convenience, at the spot or during a second reading, to satisfy your most acute curiosity, but the global 'EnjoyVity' message can be clearly understood even without consulting them.

3. 'Know how to think'

> "Happiness doesn't depend on any external conditions, it is governed by our mental attitude"   ~Dale Carnegie

It is about discovering our own strengths, authority and qualifications and purposefully using them.

Motivation: an inspirational quote, like the above, or cartoon or poster can keep you focused on a change you are trying to make in your life. Have a goal and a slogan. Print it and read aloud, repeat it daily. Take care and spend time with positive thinkers, optimists.

Discipline: once your standards are set and you decided for your action plan you should keep your focus and follow your' regime'. Find or build, strengthen that inner will power and self-discipline to overcome your weaknesses, shyness, addictions, (bad) habits, laziness and procrastination. Convince your mind that you gain inner strength when you act and DO things.
Find your examples: read how Charles Lindbergh prepared and managed to make it to Paris or how Hirotada Ototake made it in life due to his dream, discipline, motivation and optimism.

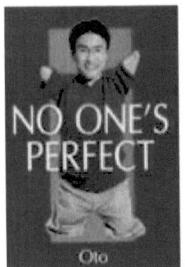 details at 'ralphmag.org/AG/ototake.html'

Psycho: includes the way you feel about yourself, the quality of your relationships, and your ability to manage your feelings and deal with difficulties. When you are mentally healthy you will be flexible to learn new things and adapt to change. Your emotional health will also help you cope when faced with life's challenges and stresses. Be open to recognize your emotions and to express them in order not to get stuck in negative moods as anxiety or depression.

Brain: masters your memory, thinking, dreaming, body-movements, metabolism,... and behavior. Well it sure is your master if it was not managed, trained and organized well from the start. Our brains are coded when we are too young to even respond to stimuli. Throughout the book you will find ways to re-program for the better your 'coding'. Repetition will be key in reprogramming your brain.

We know that "over-analysis leads to paralysis" so free your brain and **get into action**: Simplify your approach and focus on one thing at a time.

"Let me tell you the secret that has led me to my goal.
*My strength lies solely in my tenacity." ~*Louis Pasteur

How do you quiet the mind? Meditation instructors teach their students to silently repeat a mantra (a word with no meaning) repeatedly to quiet the mind. If other thoughts come to mind, you're instructed to let them pass and focus back on the mantra.

Good mental health includes the concept of **courage**, which means being willing to take action in the face of perceived danger.

> **Leave the past**
>
> **Live the now**
>
> **Enjoy the future**

Do not blame yourself, your parents, family, society or even your enemy. Society is out of balance, our civilization maybe over its top. We, Homo sapiens, are not made to live at such a pace. Our sicknesses and behavior is a result of our indecent lifestyle, rhythm and thoughts. Overeating is for many (+50% of industrialized population) a compensation for the stress assimilated on daily basis while trying to cope with workload, city life, air-, noise-, light-, water- and unseen 'electro smog'- pollution just to name these. Humans are weak don't expect miracles from others. **Not a diet is needed but a strong character able to set-up and follow a regime of positive life rules.** We cannot change this galloping complex society today, but we can change ourselves this right minute. Tomorrow you can help to change your fellowman for the better and spread hope.

It all starts NOW and with YOU!

You are the one you are waiting for. You can change!

Happiness is not in the mere possession of money; it lies in the joy of achievement, in the thrill of creative effort ~ *F.D.Roosevelt*

As we are moving into a more enlightened age:
People are already beginning to look within for the answers they seek, instead of outwards to money, possessions and other people. The more enlightened members of society will welcome the New Dawn with its emphasis on humanity, kindness, truth, spirituality and enlightenment." We are at the dawning of the Age of Aquarius, meaning we are leaving one age (Pisces), and entering into a new one (Aquarius). This happens every two thousand years. This time of crises is not the signal of the end of the world. What comes is not the end, but the beginning. The dream humanity has lived for century's ends and we awaken to a bright new day, a bright new way. ~ Shri Mataji

Do not be lost in this transition and change period. Keep it simple.
Re-become optimistic.

Attitude is the thing that keeps you young.

It is about perception
A fresh perspective
One from a position of strength, leadership and gratitude.

"If you enjoy what you do, you'll never work another day in your life."
~ Confucius

Do not get caught in the ongoing Babylonian misfiring or thinking and acting in boxes: Occidentals / Orientals, North / South, Americans / Russians, politicians / citizens, fast food / whole food, rich / poor, carnivores / vegetarians, young / old, White / Black, natives / foreigners, Catholic or Jew / Muslim, bankers / savers, nationalists/cosmopolitans, recession/boom, ...

Show the outside world **you are EnjoyVity**
Smile, laugh, eat healthy, be creative, positive, feel rich, empathic and helpful.
Grab the spirit.

"Life is a great journey through illusion. Every moment of this journey is so intense. Some people play with it, some try to learn how to win it, some just pass through it! ...I'm sinking into every passing moment. And I'm grateful for this illusion which presents me every second with a new fruit to taste: sweetness, sorrow, anger, happiness, passion and depression. All is Fullness and Emptiness. Oh, what a taste! ...I am born naked and I will die naked. All I can take from this great illusion called Life is my Spirit..." from **Naked Spirit, Sainkho.**

Do listen to Sainkho Namtchylak's extraordinary vocals on her 'Naked Spirit' CD by 'amiatamedia.com'.

Made in Africa: today the majority of goods and people are 'made in China', but not so long ago, a mere 2 million years, it was all made in East Africa, genus Homo included. So consider best relativity since we once were all black.

Indeed we "Humans" started in Africa. It may be news to Euro-Americans that they are a genetic deviation from the original dark coloration of Homo sapiens, even though in many countries today, they are dominant culturally and economically.   "If we look back only 100 or 200 generations (that's as few as 2,500 years), almost all of us were in a different place and we had a different color." ~professor Nina Jablonski, head of the Penn State Department of Anthropology

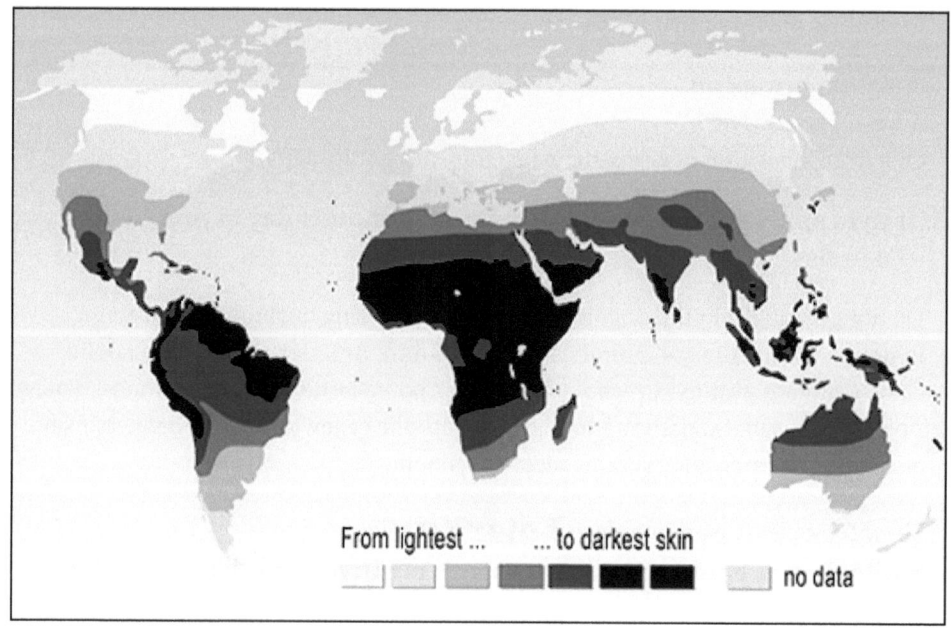

"This map shows average predicted skin color across the globe."

Source UNEP Vital Ozone Graphics, adapted from data published by George Chaplin in the *American Journal of Physical Anthropology*, Volume 125:292-302 in 2004.

Note: this book is not about religion; the bottom line remains that everybody is entitled to their beliefs.

Have a global, whole, holistic approach towards your wellbeing and wellness. Combine mind and body. Be integrated in your environment. Be 'open' minded.

No prejudices.
Inform yourself.
Ask WHY.

Step out of the more and more fictive, virtual modern world. Get that extra shock to clear your mind.

Make sure you are balanced mentally and emotionally.
Try a +3 day meditation retreat. Read(*), discuss, exercise (**) and whenever needed find confidential support and professional help.
A good place to start then on the net is 'helpguide.org'.

(*) for starters: *Meditation for Dummies*, by S.Bodian, IDG books Worldwide 1999

(**) the 'Deep Breathing' exercises, as described further in the book, are a must-do to start with

Tip: Grab 1 advice per chapter and combine towards your own personal program.

Keep the book around or find at our updated website new inspirations whenever you feel down or lost.
It happens to all of us. Sure don' think of us as Guru's (in the 'spiritual leader' sense). We only will try to show you the road to become your own Guru! Certain parts of the chapters are supporting information, other, even short sentences or quotes, may need slower reading and considering. Certain chapters might have to wait for you, as you are not ready to assimilate that information today, at this moment in your life. Give yourself time and get to the big picture then later can be in 2 months or 20 years, but you will remember ... and will come back to it.

Of course there is much more to say and write on this and on many other chapters. We just want you to find your flame and sound ground from where you start your auto-search, your self-information. As this will define the moment of REAL CHANGE IN YOU!

So remember say "No, thank you"
> to the past, depression, procrastination

> to being manipulated by the media

So remember you can add years to your life
> by controlling your stress

> by thinking positive

> by changing now

> by being "**EnjoyVity**"

4. Keep it physical

**We don't stop playing because we grow old
we grow old because we stop playing."** ~George Bernard Shaw

Exercise, stretch and move your body because moving stimulates growth, support, preservation and maintenance of the brain, healthy bone tissue, endurance, muscle mass, and strength. It helps to excrete toxins and restore balance in many of your body systems. These body systems include: the cardiovascular-, respiratory-, lymphatic-, nervous-, digestive-, reproductive-, circulatory-, urinary-, endocrine-, integumentary-(skin, hair, and nails), muscular-, skeletal- and vascular system.

You did notice that animals in nature , just as our ancestors, don't smoke, don't wear tight jeans, no synthetic panties, no high heels, no mobile phones, no alcohol, no pasteurized milk, eat everything raw, ... do deep breathing, exercise all day long and 'no-doctor'.

Exercising is very important, as you will learn throughout the book.
You should develop a plan that you can maintain permanently.
If certain exercises or habits are new to you then build your rhythm up. Start with practicing that specific exercise or idea for 60 then 120 later 180 seconds and up for instance. Or 6/12/18/24/...repetitions. Or 1/2/3/4/... exercises a day and 1/2/3/...times a day.

Repetition is 'key' in reprogramming your brain.

We will continue to help you with it at our website **'enjoyvity.com'**.
Come back regularly and send us your own stories and hints.

A man's health can be judged by which he takes two at a time - pills or stairs.
~Joan Welsh

Choose a **sweat-sport**. Run your stairs and do try some staircase workouts with Virgil Aponte at 'ultimatestairexercises.com' or at least 'tempo-walk' if you cannot run. Try Nordic walking: 'nordicwalking.com' . While walking keep your head up, look at flowers, trees, birds flying, clouds and sky. It will make you forget your worries. Set your mind free.

Don't fool yourself. Not all so-called sports are physical some are more mental like playing cards, chess or snooker. Here we talk sports which increase your heartbeat, which make you sweat.

Start with warming up then stretching, pilates or Tai-Chi, great not only for your back. Get a jump rope with digital skip counter. Lift weights for 20' three days a week, a must also while aging.

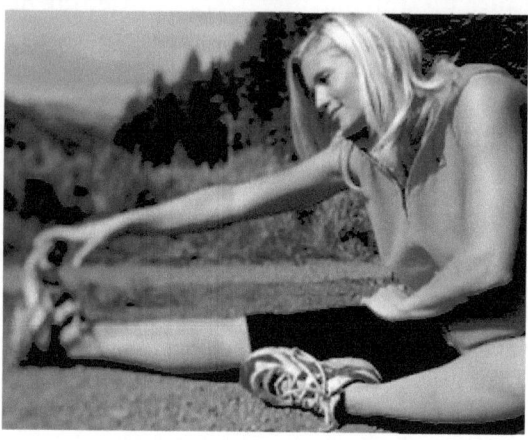

Stretching: a fundamental way to improve your overall health and fitness. In addition to improving circulation and range of motion, stretching is extremely relaxing and most users being athletes use stretching exercises to maintain a balance in body mechanics. It will improve your ability to relax and it just feels good. Have an idea how to get started while looking at good advices of an expert at fliiby.com and for many FREE examples 'myfit.ca' . See also 'Stretching for Dummies', LaReine Chabut, Wiley Publishing Inc.

Pilates: its goal is to increase the core strength of the body: the abdominal muscles, lower back and buttocks. These exercises are meant to build strength, increase flexibility and promote body and mind control. Pilates also incorporates extensive work on an exercise mat. In some respects pilates conditioning is like yoga. Both are considered mind-body type methods of movement; both emphasize deep breathing and smooth, long movements that encourage your muscles to relax and lengthen. The exercises are directly connected to **Qigong**, a 5,000-year-old Chinese exercise system. Qigong combines meditation, low-impact movements and controlled breathing to cleanse, strengthen, and circulate the life energy (qi). In China over 80 million persons are doing Qigong. Check it at 'jsqg.sport.org.cn' and for many FREE Pilates exercises 'myfit.ca' or extra information at 'pilates-method-exercise.com'.

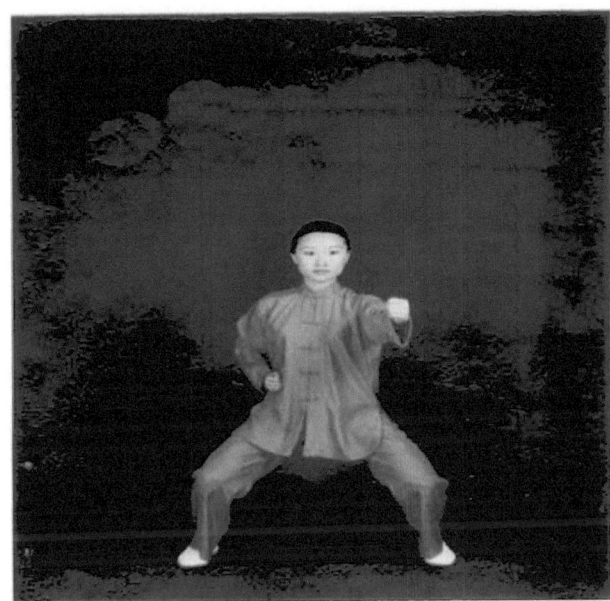

QiGong Routine 7 to enhance strength

It's almost impossible to describe how to do a **Tai-Chi chuan** '<u>slow</u>' movement correctly—you really need to see someone else doing it to understand. The best way to it is from an instructor, classes tend to be relatively inexpensive. Specialized medical advisers have documented that Tai-Chi helps improve posture, reduce spinal degeneration, maintain flexibility of joints, improve balance, and increase strength and stability in the lower back. Also here it all starts with correct breathing as we will learn you later. Let the energy and love stream through your body.

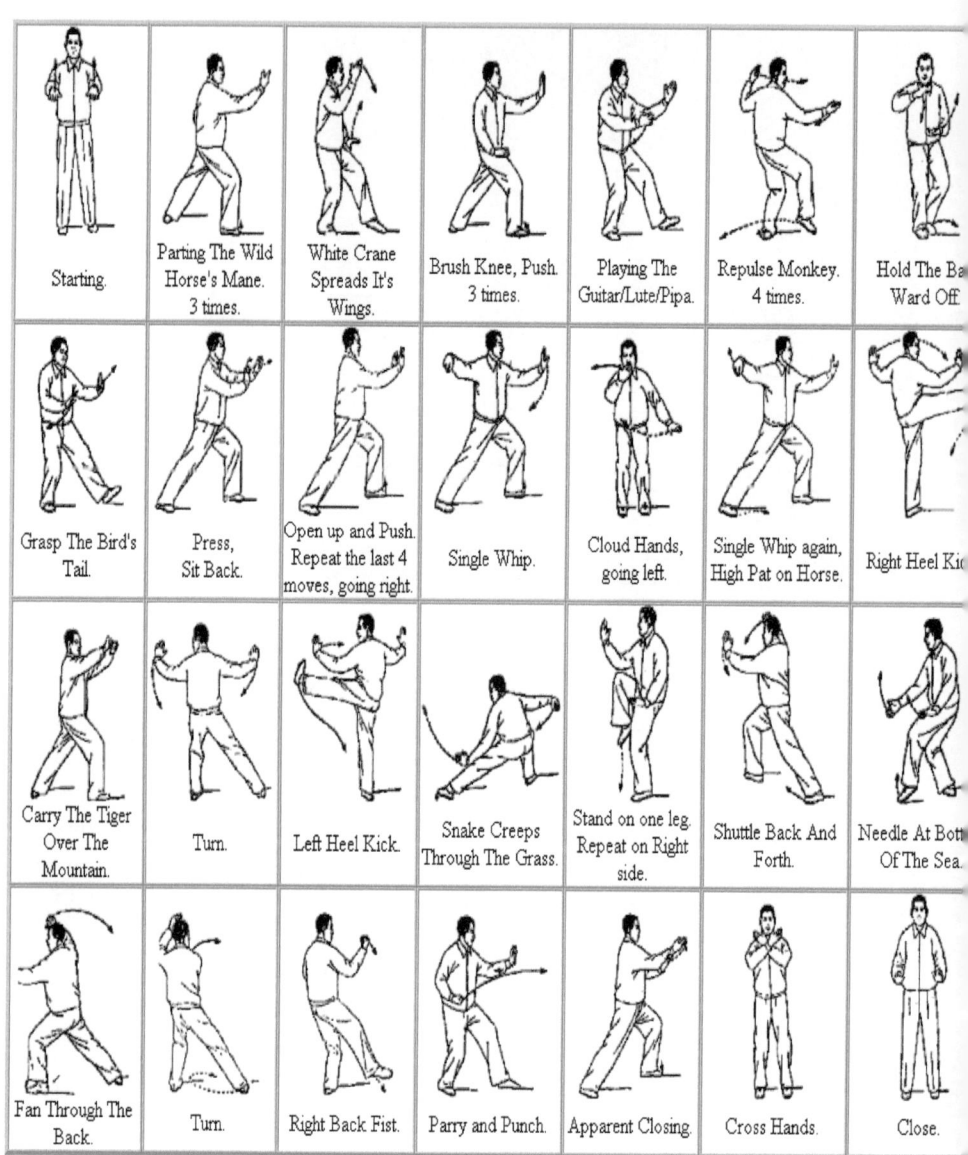

Get finally or again physical, move your skeleton, put a smile and start sweating the rewards will be yours only. Gardening is fun, but not a sport these days with all the motorized engines we use. Switch back from the self-tracking grass mower or worse the modern tractor with a seat and turn it in a healthy exercise again. Just wash your car by hand and burn those calories while saving $$. You will feel excited afterwards knowing that you did 3 important things at once. Good for your self-esteem.

Some soft exercises:

1. **The 'Zero-Neck-Roll'** (*): move your head

    a. forward/backward: close your eyes and effortlessly and gently let your head drop forward and backward (stretch two seconds while in this position for extra de-stress), then again forward and backward. Do each exercise four times to begin with. Later on you can increase the number to six or more. When dropping the head backward keep your facial muscles relaxed; the lips should part slightly when the head is thrown back.

    b. turn head extreme left/then right: while turning the head to the sides contracts the muscles, returning to normal position relaxes them.

    c. bend left/right: move ear to your shoulder

    d. neck out/in: resembles the neck movements of a turtle, for you should literally "stick your neck out" as far as you can, then draw it back again

Benefits of these neck exercises: Improve vitality, sleep, vision and hearing and prevent headaches, since the nerves and blood vessels in the neck go to the head and brain. Great thus to start the morning and finish the evening or before start learning, reading, working, driving, ... see also 'holisticonline.com'

(*) the classical 360 degree neck roll brings stress to your neck joints which can lead to inflammation

2. Use some **unknown muscles**: now and then walk with your basin and pubis area turned forward it will tighten your butt and make you burn more calories than when not doing so. Also because you will make shorter steps and thus move more and probably faster over the same distance. You can laugh while doing so. Only the result counts, try it.

3. The **Cobra** posture one out of many great, balancing yoga poses:

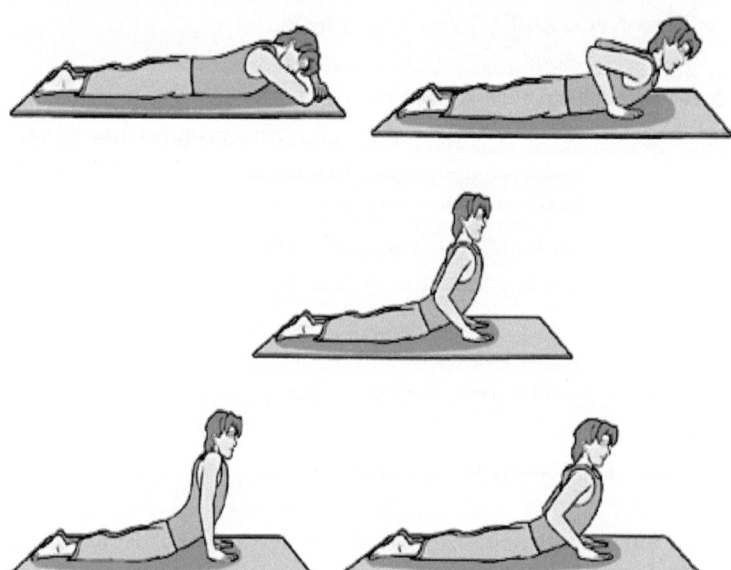

It will bring you a multiple of benefits as it is a great exercise for people with lower back aches. This posture decreases stiffness in the lower back, enlarges the chest, and strengthens the arms and shoulders. The posture is also good to combat menstrual irregularities, and it helps relieve stress.
For a dynamic visualization: 'abc-of-yoga.com' and for the original approach start at 'india-shopping.net' under related topics you will find tons of information to improve your body and mind flexibility.

4) the **Thorax** increaser: while sitting on a chair press with hands your knees together, or while walking press your hands against your hips. Now 'stomach'-breathe IN from the nose till the maximum with 'shocks'. Keep your breath. Slowly, but completely, breathe OUT through the mouth, again with repetitive shocks while keeping your lips tightly together. This exercise will increase your thorax volume drastically if repeated for months. It will fight overwrought, stress, irritability and let vanish all fatigue.

Reach for the extreme and learn about your limits.

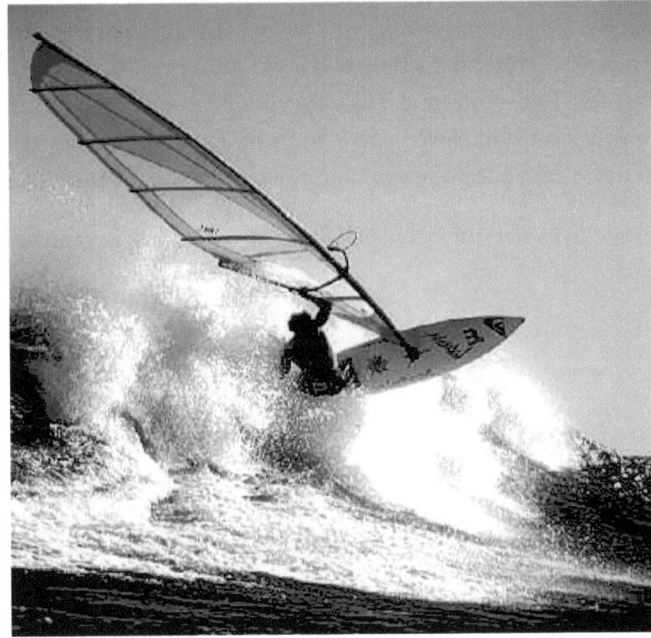

Explode now and then.

Dare to go beyond. Make a Bungee jump. Don't know where, no problem: 'bungeezone.com'

Your safe(r) adrenaline: Ballooning, dancing, windsurf, paraglide ('paraglide.com'), fishing, hiking or bear watching in Siberia ('naturetrek.co.uk'). Find your thrill sport at '1001sportsworld.blogspot.com' . At best start **rowing**!

Or just have a dawn **dew walk** in spring and listen to your body and the surrounding nature. It stimulates your whole body through the reflex points on your foot sole and your blood circulation and overall awareness. Stepping on naked feet in the dewed grass, acts as a strong reducing agent or anti-oxidant and will de-stress many in minutes. Stay connected!

Weight training is especially important: you should be "really' building muscle on daily base! Lifting weights helps maintain bone density and also lessens the risk of falls at any age.

Build muscles not fat: Losing a lot of fat and gaining a lot of muscle at the same time is very hard to do. Your body will decide if it makes first muscles or releases fat. It only takes 15 extra grams of protein a day to build a pound of muscle a week -- so you really won't need to eat a lot more. Muscle takes much less volume than fat. So stay motivated and measure up. If you are inactive, you lose muscle mass to the point where you are unable to carry out daily activities -- climbing stairs, getting up out of a chair -- because your muscles are not strong enough to move the weight of your own body. Don't try to add fat to a weak body. Just start an exercise program and build muscles. Strength training will build muscle while decreasing step by step your body fat. Take your time, evaluate after 8 weeks. Eating healthy will further decrease your body fat. Never starve yourself. Fat is emergency storage for your body. If you don't eat your body will hold the fat and burn muscles.

Lack of physical exercise ages not only your body, but also your brain. Step away from your PC ...

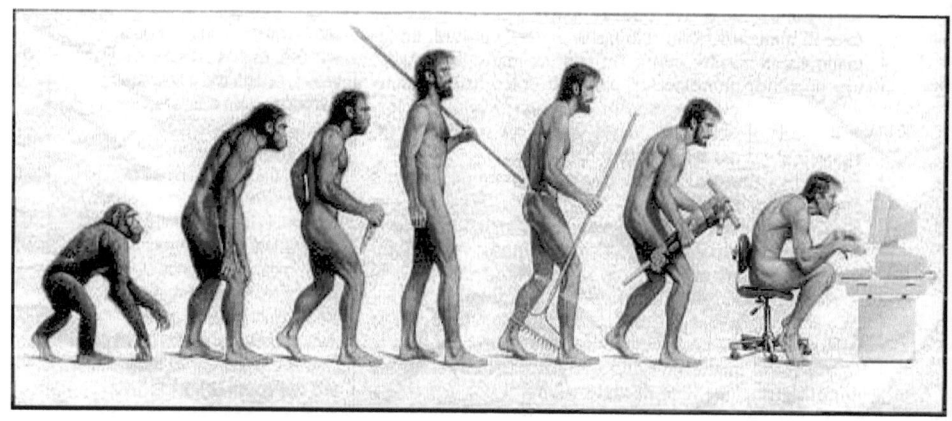

Somewhere, something went terribly wrong

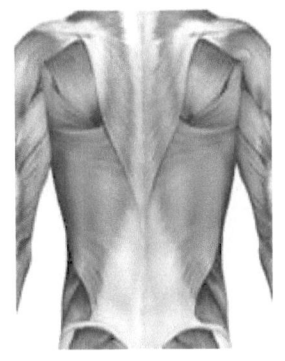 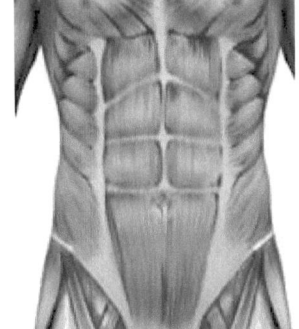 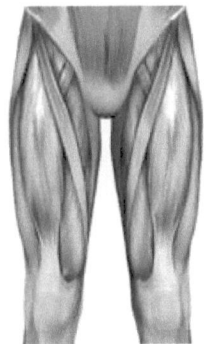

Build Muscles start now, get advice: 'myfit.ca'

If you are over 40 and have never before exercised, be sure to check with your doctor before beginning an intensive exercise program.

So remember say "No, thank you"
> to laziness

> to PC craziness

So remember you can add years to your life

> by breathing correctly

> by exercising

> by acting "**EnjoyVity**"

This information is not intended to be a substitute for professional medical care, and is presented as information **only**.

5. Know how and what to eat

"If you think we are meat-eaters then try eating the animal raw like every other meat-eater on the planet. If something is not palatable in its raw state then you probably shouldn't be eating it."   ~*David Wolfe*

In order to maintain one's health and organ structure a human consumes approximately **50 Ton of food** during the course of a lifetime. You better make the right choice!

Our food and eating habits are important. For 99.9% of human existence, our predecessors lived for millions of years on foods that were either raw or minimally processed: fruits, vegetables, meats, nuts and seeds. The technology needed to increase food processing did not exist until very recently.   Most of us eat in a totally different way as our parents or grandparents and not always for the better. Let's zoom in, as the saying goes: **"You are what you Eat"**

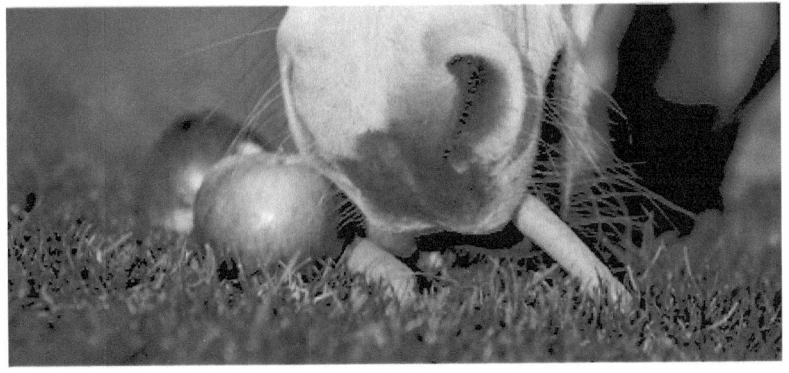

What does it then mean *he eats like a horse*? Horses will never over-eat.

Or *she eats like a pig*! This slim girl wants truffles!

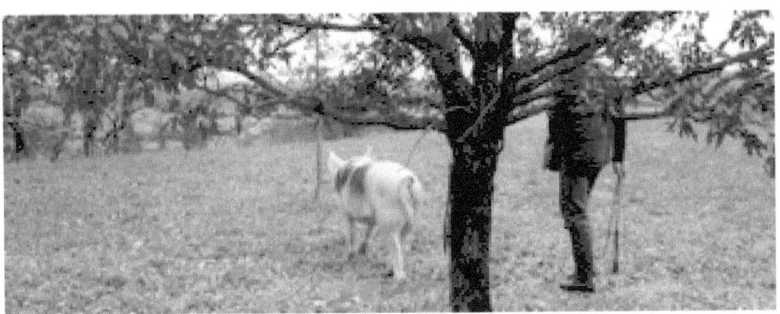

Find me a corpulent horse or wild boar! I can find you a condominium-cat or house-dog with obesity easily.

How come? Overeating of canned or processed food and not enough exercise, maybe?

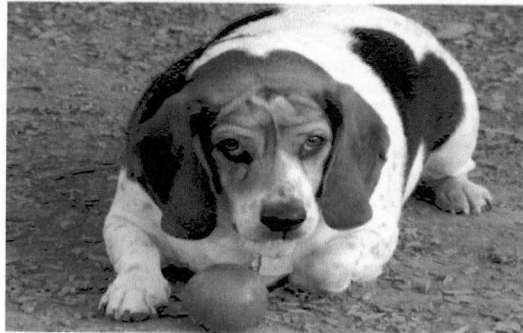

Find me a fat fox at a leach.

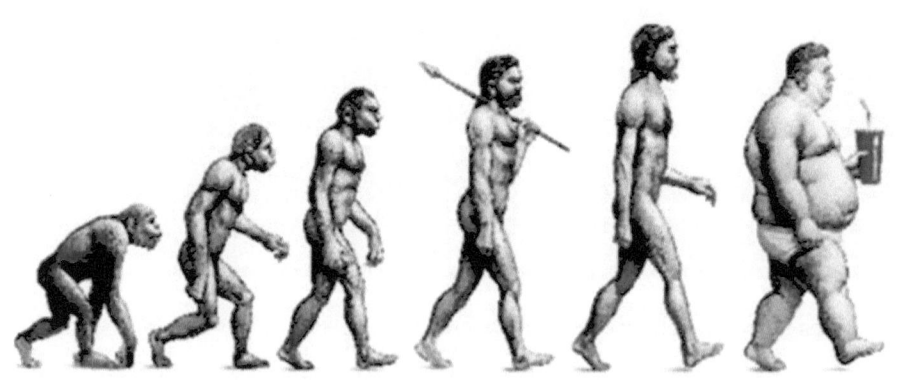

"The shape of things to come!" ~*The Economist* 12-11-2003

Initially **'homo sapiens'** was a hunter-gatherer (*) who tried to subsist in a wild environment with a scarcity of food, since 10.000 years with the emergence of agriculture relative abundance came with still cycles of feast and famine to which man was adapted. Our modern western diet and lifestyle, in place since less than 100 years and characterized by abundance of processed foods, is creating nutritional disorders, decrease in muscle mass and increase in fat mass. While many countries, not to say billions of people, in our world have endemic starvation those who could escape to the western society and assimilate these diets, lifestyles and habits, suffer from the same chronic '**epidemical**' diseases like, but not only obesity, within a generation. (*)Our ancestors ate meat and lots of vegetables, but no grains (*bread, donuts, rice, pasta ...*).

We are not showing you the 1001-th **miracle diet**. We will not guide you from excesses (mal-nutrition, overeating) to new extremes which bring your immune system down and make you jump back once you dare to stop that specific (low calorie) approach. **We at "EnjoyVity" are opting with our holistic vision for a total, balanced, body and mind program;** respecting your whole person, including your true physical, nutritional, and lifestyle needs.

Anyhow the latest most profound study *Comparison of Weight-Loss Diets with Different Compositions of Fat, Protein, and Carbohydrates* (*) can best be summarized as: 'Four Low-Calorie Diets Yield the Same Mediocre Results.'(*) ~Dr. Frank Sacks &Co, a professor at the Harvard School of Public Health, New England Journal of Medicine, 02-2009. Furthermore are nutrition scientists getting aware, at least in-door, that dieting is more a question of change in behavior rather than of actual food composition.

Eating just like living 'right' should not be more expensive.
Learn to eat less, but more whole, balanced and live healthier.

Choose and prepare your eating environment and party. Eat in a relaxed atmosphere whenever possible. No mobiles. Do not eat if you are not in the mood, if you are not hungry or have no time.
Eat fresh and seasonal. Not just an expression, but one which might bring a total change in your eating habits. Think it over!

Chew **30 times**: meaning after biting with your incisors use your molars thoroughly for grinding. If you cannot make it till even 10 times, then question your eating habits (rushing with all others maybe) and what you are eating (too refined probably); mixing and digestion should start in your mouth as your **saliva contains specific rich enzymes** (*) for it and your stomach has not a 500 RPM chopping function as your kitchen blender does and which you can crank up to 20,000 RPM to liquefy ingredients in seconds. The longer food stays in the mouth being chewed, the stronger the signal to the stomach and pancreas to start releasing the appropriate enzymes to facilitate the digestion.
(*) Find more on enzymes under chapter 8.
The process of eating should be mouthwatering, try it out 'literally'. Take just one larger nut, for instance a 'Macadamia,' chew on it 10, 20 till 30 times, mix with your saliva. Possible right! Now continue an extra 10 times or more if you start liking it. Noticed the difference between what you had in your mouth after 5 or 10 teeth

bites or after 35 grinds and chewing? Understand now better about pre-digestion, assimilation and health.

You still think it is time consuming or a waist? If so, start then with the right amount, you will compensate. Eat less. Split an entrée with a friend. Take portions the size of your fist or ones you should be able to cover with your hand. Use your 5 senses fully to enjoy every bite. Look in your plate, listen your teeth, smell what is on your fork, feel the food on your lips and taste it with your tongue. Give some eye sparkles to your meal partner and enjoy.

Start with the right smallest possible plate or take half portions and no second ones. Portions are oversized these days. Are you sure that your dog needs this bag with leftovers? Eating slowly, research suggests, can encourage people to eat less, and enjoy the meal more. The reason is that it takes about 20 minutes for our brains to register that we're full. If we eat fast, we can continue eating past the point where we are full.

Go for quality not quantity and enjoy.

Maybe just read this section again as for most of us it is a big piece of the puzzle of life. It will take less than a minute even less than half a minute for "fast-readers".

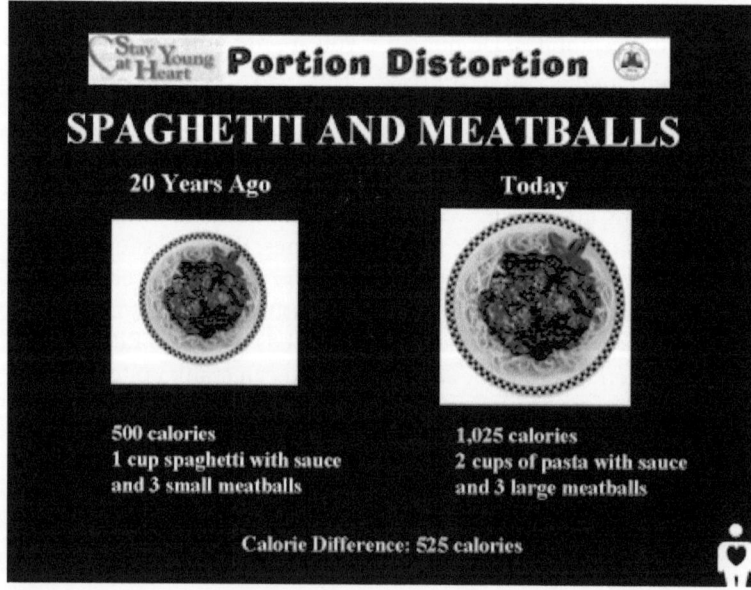

More than double the calories in 20 years! Look also at the difference in the plate sizes!

Try not to eat while working, driving or when you are otherwise on the go.
Find that time, like monks, they still eat in silence to fully appreciate their plate's content.
Make that time, use a table or dessert spoon to savor your fresh vegetable soup. Business lunches or dinners are rather unhealthy as they leave little time for smelling, tasting not to say chewing correctly. Many times participants at a business lunch don't even remember what they were eating exactly.

Our Food should be Bio, Eco and green at first.
And colorful, diverse, less cooked and prepared for sure. It is about feeding your 600 trillion of cells (read details chapter 8).

Katherine Tucker, professor of nutritional epidemiology at Tufts University, states" The relationship between cardiovascular disease and **prevention** in epidemiological studies is stronger for the intake of fruit and vegetables than for any kind of mineral or vitamin supplement."

The Food Pyramid: there are many in circulation and **under ongoing discussion** (*); For the moment I prefer the one from the University of Michigan (**) because it clearly shows that the base of everything is WATER, lots of healthy water daily, followed by fresh FRUIT and fresh VEGETABLES. At best to be overlaid with the latest one of Doctor Walter C. Willett and Co. at the Harvard School of public health who add correctly at the base 'daily exercise and weight control' and many other healthy advices(*). Give it a look at **'harvard.edu';** where you can also download a larger image of 'The Healthy Eating Pyramid'. Note that Doctor Willet's team research does **not confirm at all** the **'low fat is good health'** message!
(*) such as: Easily digested carbohydrates from white bread, white rice, pastries, sugared sodas, and other highly processed foods may contribute to weight gain, interfere with weight loss, and promote diabetes and heart disease.

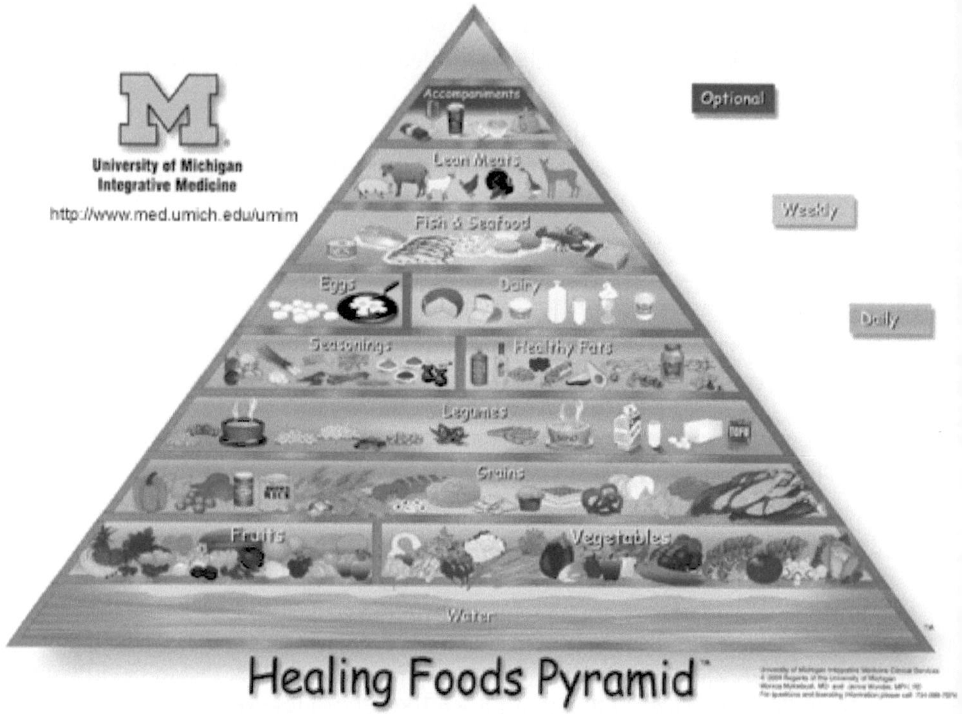

Healing Foods Pyramid

If you go online here 'med.umich.edu' you can get all details while clicking on each segment of the pyramid, start from the bottom with a glass or 2 of pure water. Also educational is 'mypyramid.gov'

(*) **Discussion:** Read for instance "Cereal Killer" of Alan L. Watson; check out 'modern-diets-and-nutritional-diseases.com' and 'westonaprice.org' so you understand the importance of words like 'lean', 'raw' and 'full' and the controversy between traditional ways of food and nutrition and modern sources of food manufacturing.

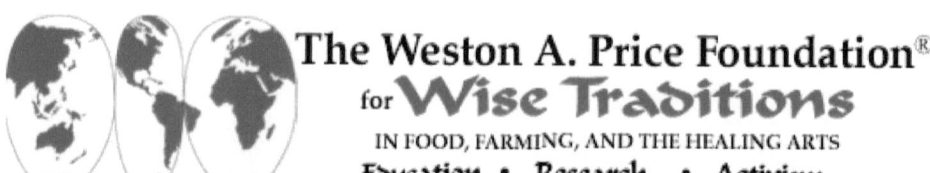

(**)The University of Michigan Integrative Medicine Clinical Services. Their mission is to care for people using an **Integrative Medicine** model that reaffirms the importance of relationship between practitioner and patient, focuses on the whole person, is informed by evidence, and makes use of all appropriate therapeutic approaches **to achieve optimal health and healing.**

> The Institute of Medicine recommends that adults get a minimum of 0.8 grams of **protein** for every kilogram of body weight per day—that's about 60 grams for a 160 pound (70 kilo) adult. Probably much less than you actually are eating. Check it out.

Average Calorie intake through time and age:

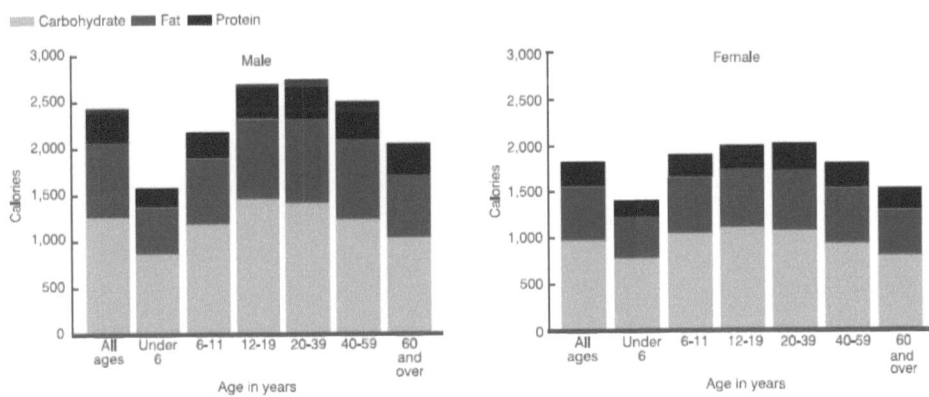

Figure 1. Total calorie intake and major sources of calories for U.S. population, NHANES 1999-2000

In the USA: "During 1971- 2000, a statistically significant increase in average energy intake occurred. For men, average energy intake increased from 2,450 to 2,618 kcals, and for women, from 1,542 to 1,877 kcals." The rest of the industrialized countries follow in these steps. What is happening in the rest of the world is shown in this table:

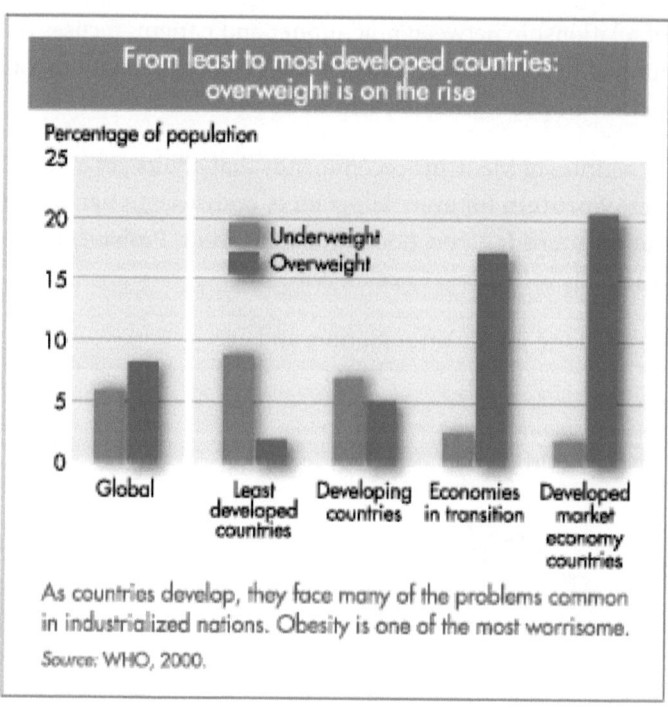

As countries develop, they face many of the problems common in industrialized nations. Obesity is one of the most worrisome.
Source: WHO, 2000.

Obesity is thus clearly and mainly a modern disease which now even touches our young children for whom it might be an irreversible process. The prevalence of obesity (BMI≥30) continues to be a health concern for adults, children and adolescents in the United States. Data from the most recent NHANES survey shows that among adult men the prevalence of obesity grew to 33.3% in 2005—2006 and to 35.3% for woman.

Another recent NHANES survey found that among children and adolescents aged 2-19 years 16.3% were obese. See also the USA-Statistics page ~226.

In past centuries the working class was slim and the bureaucrats opulent. As until recently, only the wealthiest people could afford to feed, raise, and slaughter animals for their flesh. Consequently, prior to the 20th century, only the rich died from diseases like heart disease, obesity, and strokes.

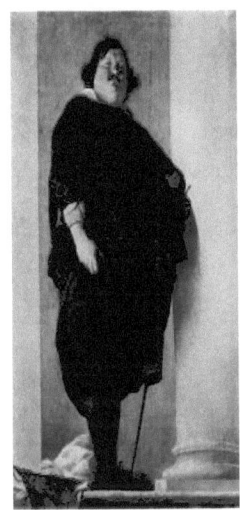
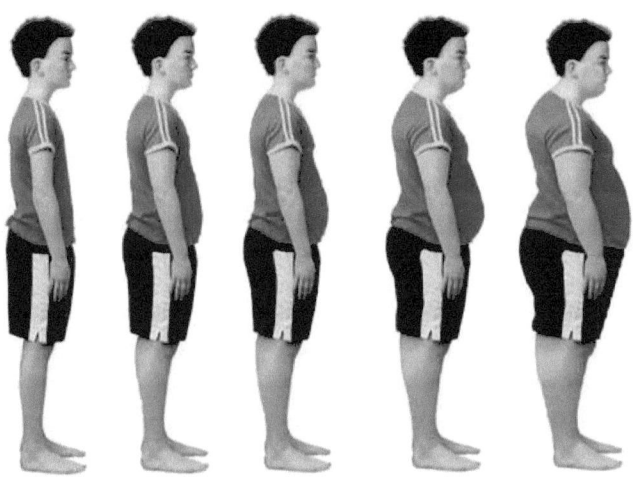

Today the intelligent and rich minority is slim and the average citizen has more than less overweight. We are sure you have an idea why.

The World Health Organization (WHO) classifies about 400 million people around the world as obese, and the numbers are increasing.

Are your friends making you fat? Or keeping you slender? According to new research from Harvard and the University of California, San Diego, the short answer on both counts is "yes".

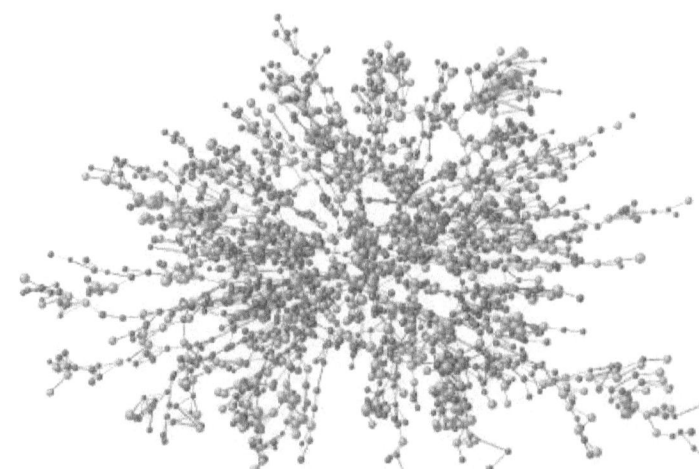

A social network map of 2,200 people, the largest group of connected individuals in the Framingham

Heart Study, in the year 2000. Each circle represents one person, and the size of each circle is proportional to that person's body-mass index (BMI). Yellow circles indicate people who are considered medically obese and green circles indicate people who are not obese. Lines indicate family and friendship ties. (Credit: Figure courtesy of James Fowler, UC San Diego (2007, July 26). Obesity Is 'Socially Contagious')

So remember that your social circle should be supportive to your 'new' lifestyle. Surround yourself with healthy and balanced people, or at least help and try to turn 'unbalanced' over.

"What smoking was to my parents' generation, obesity is to my children's generation."
~David Paterson Governor N.Y. (defender of an 'obesity tax' on soft drinks)

The **surgeon general** estimates that obesity was associated with 112,000 deaths in the United States <u>every year</u>.

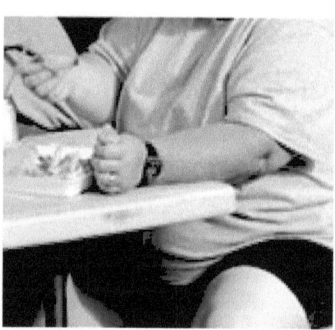 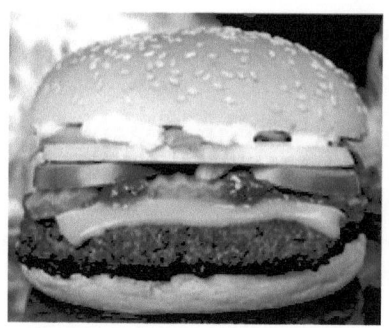

The obesity epidemic is not confined to the USA; similar increases are being seen worldwide as other countries adopt Western high-calorie foods and a sedentary lifestyle. The National Statistics Office in Korea, for example, indicate that nearly a third of Koreans (about 10 million people) are overweight, with numbers increasing by about 400,000 annually.

> Grab the source of the problem rather than to seek a quick fix.
> Understand that drinking diet colas with your super-sized bag of chips is not a good idea.

Remove the industrially-processed (refined, canned, treated *) foods from your meals and snacks and your body will normalize. Metabolism, hormonal systems and weight will become normal.

Say No to processed food: it is easy, if it has more than 6 ingredients in it - don't eat it. If it has anything that you cannot pronounce or don't know what it is - don't eat it.

* **some examples of processed foods:** margarine and shortening, pizza, fast foods, fried foods like French fries and fried chicken, doughnuts, cookies, sweets, pastries, crackers, processed foods like cereal and waffles, salad dressings, mayonnaise, chips, convenience foods, canned foods,....
Most of them are ready to eat (or just need microwave heating) and have a LONG shelf life. Read more: 'healthy-eating-politics.com'.

What is in it now which was not then? Check these **additive** list: 'cspinet.org' or with E-numbering 'food.gov.uk'.

Ninety percent of Americans' household food budget is spent on processed foods, the majority of which are filled with additives and stripped of nutrients.
Today, half of the United States food budget is used to buy food at restaurants.

How Come? Due to industrialization and urbanization and while at more and more families both partners work outside there is less or no time left for traditional food preparation. So fast food, pre-packed and processed foods are a help or must for many. Then due to the marketing machine! The fast food industry spends close to $11 billion/year promoting their products while the US Government spends 3% of that amount for 'healthy living' promotion. Need extra motivation read 'Fatal Harvest': 'fatalharvest.org' or Rachel Carson's 'Silent Spring': 'rachelcarson.org'

MUFA, PUFA, SFA, TFA and even Inter**ester**ified ? *The confusion* is all about fats and oils. Most treated foods have mixed quantities of the first 3.
At the turn of the 19th century Americans consumed less than one (1!) pound a year of liquid vegetable oil and 100 years later at the close of the 20th century they were consuming over 75 pounds per year of highly processed vegetable oil.
Scientists are still arguing about fat, despite a century of research, because the regulation of appetite and weight in the human body happens to be almost inconceivably complex, and the experimental tools we have to study it are still remarkably inadequate.
Omega-3 and omega-6 fatty acids are types of **PUFA** and are considered essential fatty acids because our bodies cannot make them, thus they must be obtained through the diet. They provide antioxidants such as vitamin E and selenium. Some research suggests that diets including **MUFA** (like olive oil) can have a positive effect on cholesterol, blood pressure, blood clotting and inflammation.
NO to saturated- and trans-fats (SFA or TFA)!? As 'the medical community' say they increase your cholesterol levels. Although, ask a specialist and insider, Dr.

Dwight Lundell, cardiovascular surgeon: *"Inflammation Is the real reason Over 850,000 people die every year from heart disease!" Get informed:* 'thecholesterol-lie.com'

Conjugated linoleic acids (CLA), what!? It's a family of isomers of linoleic acids found especially in meat and dairy products, highly in the news due to their anti-oxidants and anti-cancer properties. Of all foods, kangaroo meat may have the highest concentration of CLA. Food products from **grass-fed beef** and other ruminants are good sources of CLA. In fact, meat and dairy products from grass-fed animals can produce 300-500% more CLA than those of cattle fed the usual diet of 50% hay and silage, and 50% grain. CLA recently is attributed too many health benefits (*) and many people started taking CLA as an expensive supplement. (*) increasing metabolic rate, decreasing abdominal fat, enhancing muscle growth up to enhancing the immune system. Follow the discussion and meanwhile find your CLA's in **naturally grown products** like in cheese made from milk from **grass fed** cows, as it will also have higher levels of calcium, proteins, beta-carotene, vitamin A, vitamin D, and vitamin E and a perfect healthy balance of omega 3 and 6, or from Australian pastoral lamb meat or kangaroo. Stay informed get a second opinion like from Dr. Mercola: 'mercola.com'

The importance of **balancing omega 3 and omega 6 fats:** our omega 6 intake has doubled from what it was in 1940 and our intake of omega 3 fatty acids has shrunk to one sixth of 1850 levels! Today the average western diet is thus too high in omega-6 (lineolic acid or **LA**) and dangerously low in Omega-3 (Alpha-Linolenic Acid or **ALA** from plant food sources(*)). It is not a matter of 6 is bad and 3 is good, it is the balance of the two in relation to each other which is key. The two fatty acids work differently in the metabolism and are in a synergy - so try to keep them within a balance **2:1** is the best ratio of Omega-3 & -6 fatty acids. Over-dominance of omega-6 creates a situation ('terrain') that can cause increased water retention, raised blood pressure and blood clotting and promotes chronic inflammation, cancer propagation, diabetes, arthritis and heart diseases. Omega-3 fatty acids improve cholesterol levels and reduce heart attack and stroke. **Omega-9**'s are found in animal fats and vegetable oils, most notably olive oil. Interestingly, the oil made by our skin glands is the same omega-9 fatty acid found abundantly in olive oil: oleic acid.   (*) active ingredients in omega 3 are named **EPA** (Eicosapentaenoic Acid) and **DHA** (Docosahexaenoic Acid) when from animal mainly fish source.

In the last 50 years our way of food preparing and eating changed to the extent that many of our foods are now **fried** in vegetable oils. In traditional cooking, foods were boiled, baked or roasted.

If we get the right kind of fats in the right and balanced amounts and prepared using the right methods, they will build our health and keep us healthy.

Table of major fatty acids		
Omega-3 fatty acids *polyunsaturated* (PUFA's)	**Omega-6 fatty acids** *polyunsaturated* (PUFA's)	**Omega-9 fatty acids** *monounsaturated* (MUFA's)
Alpha linolenic acid (ALA, or more commonly LNA) — *essential*	Linoleic acid (**LA**) — *essential*	Oleic acid
Eicosapentaenoic acid (**EPA**)	Gamma-linolenic acid (**GLA**)	Mead acid
Docosahexaenoic acid (**DHA**)	Arachidonic acid (**AA**)	Erucic acid

Balancing is also 'keep change' in your **cooking and dressing oils** to supply the body with all types of necessary nutrients and a balanced omega 3 and 6 quotient.

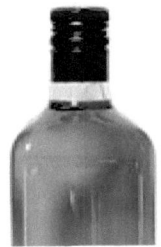

Choose from and **switch** between: rapeseed oil, flaxseed oil (not for cooking as heat sensitive), walnut oil, virgin olive oil, soya oil, corn oil, sunflower oil, sesame oil, coconut oil, oat-germ oil, safflower oil, canola oil, palm kernel oil, argan oil, cashew oil, pumpkin seed oil, krill oil, macadamia nut oil, cocoa butter... or better use your own favorite mixture.

DIVERSIFICATION! Your body will appreciate and decide for itself what building blocks it needs at every moment.

Re-introducing foods rich in omega-3 fatty acids will automatically counterbalance the over-usage of omega-6 rich foods. Salmon, sardines, tuna, anchovy, cod, cod liver oil, scallops, flax seeds (ground them for improved assimilation), oregano, cauliflower, broccoli, cabbage (as most dark green leafy vegetables) and walnuts are excellent food sources of omega 3 fatty acids. Vitamin E, the primary fat-soluble antioxidant, protects omega 3 fats from oxidation. Choosing the right foods and bringing variety in your meals will not only keep it interesting and inspiring for everyone around the table, but also balance your overall vitamin, fat, protein, carbohydrates, fibers, ... intake and decrease the need for supplements. All types of lean and fatty meats are part of this balanced approach. Cooking should be FUN and it starts with enjoying the shopping for it.

Omega-3 in Fresh or Frozen Fish

Type of fish	mg/100 g
Roe, mixed	2 354
Mackerel (Atlantic Ocean)	2 299
Herring (Pacific Ocean)	1 658
Herring (Atlantic Ocean)	1 571
Mackerel (Pacific Ocean)	1 441
Black cod	1 395
Salmon (Pacific Ocean)	1 355
Mackerel, Spanish	1 341
White fish, mixed	1 258
Tuna, bluefin	1 173
Salmon, red	1 172
Pink salmon	1 005

Source: U.S. Department of Agriculture

Fish oil: known for greatly reducing inflammation in our body, which reverses the effects of aging and ensures a healthy heart, brain, joints, digestive and immune system. You can eat fatty fish or use fish oils to get these beneficial effects. Eating fish will not provide the levels of nutrients that are found in cod liver oil. Even in heavy fish-eating populations, the addition of cod liver oil improves health. **Cod liver oil** contains extra vitamins D next to vitamins A and is advisable in sun restricted areas or seasons. The top is **krill** (small shrimp)oil with the highest antioxidant properties (300x of fish oil).Fish-, krill- and cod liver oil from a high quality source don't pose the same potential risk of contamination with heavy metals and toxic chemicals as fresh fish, because they are purified of mercury, PCBs and many other contaminants.

Meat and dairy products will contain omega-3 but the animals must then have been fed fresh grass, something which is not so common today with the demand for high productivity. Cows eating grain produce more milk, but the milk will contain less omega-3s and other nutrients.

Make the right choices, buy foods where hydrogenated and partially hydrogenated vegetable oils are not listed as ingredients.
Prefer fresh, raw and steamed cooking with organic veggies and grass fed meat of your choice. Read also 'Organic, Inc.' ~ Samuel Fromartz, and understand about your power as consumer; 'fromartz.com' and check out: 'whfoods.com'.

We must REPEAT choose for **MODERATION**, balanced, seasonal and whole foods. While 'whole' means 'not' refined. So say NO, THANK YOU to all bread products made of whitened flour which contains 'alloxan', a disaster for our pancreas. More information on this and other related topics: 'naturalnews.com'.

Same for **fried foods**: NO!
OK, once a week or better a month then, as the exception should make the rule also here. Indeed, food is a great source of pleasure, and pleasure is good for the heart – even if those 'Belgian' fries aren't!

> If after reading part, most or all of the here set out information, you agree that the *EnjoyVity* approach is doable, holistic and the one to spread, than do so.

Why do so many people gain weight in midlife?
Blame it on hormones in convergence with poor lifestyle choices, overeating, not exercising enough, and stress (read emotions). But hormones only account for about 2 to 5 pounds (1 to 2,5 kilo).

Where am I: Calculate your BMI (Body Mass Index):

English BMI Formula BMI = (Weight in Pounds / (Height in inches) x (Height in inches)) x 703

Metric BMI Formula BMI = (Weight in Kilograms / (Height in Meters) x (Height in Meters))

BMI Categories for people between 18 and 65 years:

- Underweight = 18.5 or less
- Normal weight = 18.5-24.9
- Overweight = 25-29.9
- Obesity = BMI of 30 or greater (with 40 or greater reflecting a Morbid Obesity)

'cdc.gov' or at our site 'enjoyvity.com/bmi'.

Even during a weight control program you and your friends are not really interested in your weight, but in your measurements, your silhouette.
So throw away your balance and use your ribbon meter to measure up your belly. As even with a normal BMI you can have visual concerns about your figure.
Good to know that grease is much lighter (thus takes more volume) than your bones or muscles. Also while changing eating and moving habits you might exchange grease for muscles which reflects not always in a weight change but definitely in a change for the better of your silhouette.

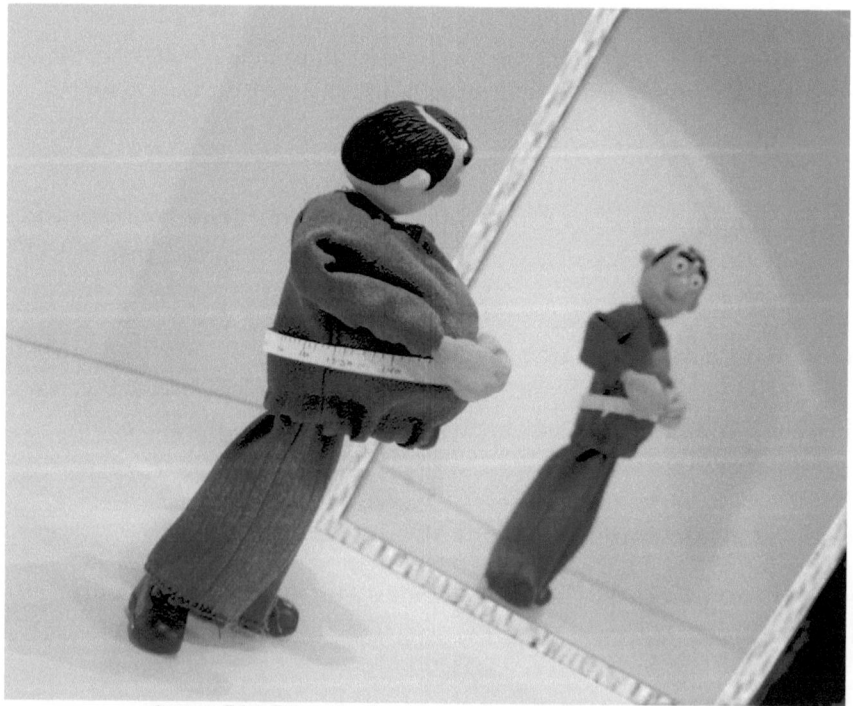

Courtesy Dépt. Prévention-Santé Prov de Luxembourg

Note down, what is today ....your BMI .... your Waist circumference ....cm/inch. Your goal........cm/inch.

Measure-up your waist:
Waist line for men less than 102 cm / 40" and 89 cm / 35" for woman, better even when less than 94/37" for men and 80/31.5" for woman. There is an optimal weight and thus look or volume for every-body and which will differ in function of height, age, constitution or shape. Some genetically defined shapes can't be changed without chirurgical help. Some overweight people have stored their excess body fat in the upper body, the apple types, easier to get rid off than the fat stored in the lower body, the pear types. The further you are from that optimum the slower you should move up or back to reach it. Since the majority of people are overweight here an example.

Take **10% motivational steps** on monthly, bimonthly or even longer time towards your optimal goal. Say your BMI is 30 and your waist line+133 cm/52.4" so as a man you are 41cm/16.2" of your optimum waist line target (92cm/36.2"). First step is to bring it down by just 5cm/2" in 4 weeks, no harm if it takes you 6 or 8 (*). Then you cover the remaining gap of 36cm/14.1" by 4cm/1.57" steps during the 2nd till the 4th step. From the 5th month or step on you decrease your intermediate target to 3cm/1.18" and later till 2cm/0.78" and even 1cm/0.4" to reach your master-target. Evaluate not after 10 weeks but 10 months.
(*) following your combination of our advices throughout the book might move you much faster down the line.

Your BMI is over 30. Please continue reading and set NOW an appointment with your physician, psychologist or anyone you are accepting and trusting to be capable to motivate you towards your healthy way out.

Being overweight and staying that way is not good for your health and longevity, not to mention your wallet, once those medical expenses for drugs and surgery start to roll in.
Burning excess calories is not that easy: 500 calories (equals 2 small pizza slices, like 25 years ago) needs 4 miles (+6,4 km) of running or walk 1hour and 10 minutes for a 153 pounder (+70 kg); take care, the today 2 large slices will bring 850 calories!

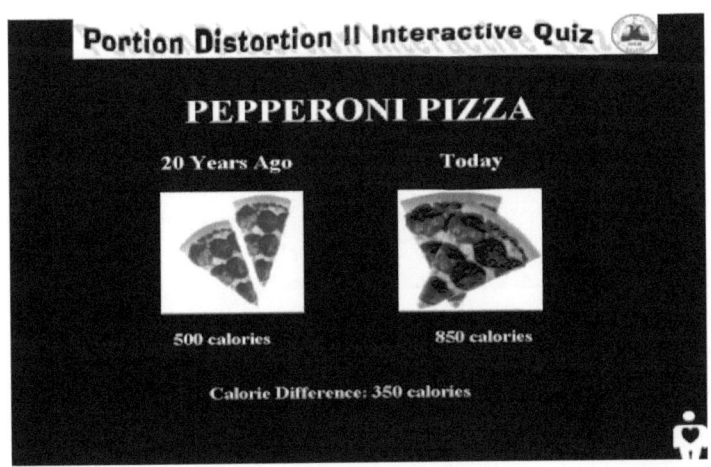

It takes over 45' of tennis to burn the extra 350 calories and even more than **2 hours** of aerobic dance to burn these 850 calories!

Extra motivation: scientists in California found that middle-aged people who run 40' a day, for a total of about 5 hours per week — lived longer and functioned better physically and cognitively as they got older.

Better to **avoid those extra daily calories** or at least understand how to burn them: to burn 165 calories it takes 35 minutes of garden work or walking or 17 minutes of brisk-walking (5MPH/8km/hr) or 17 minutes of moderate crow swimming or 17 minutes of leisure biking and almost 100 minutes of computer work.

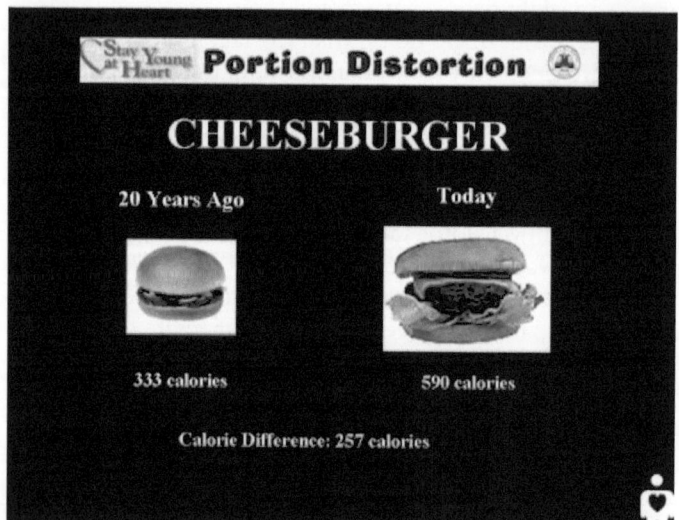

Calculate for yourself: 'primusweb.com' and 'caloriesperhour.com'

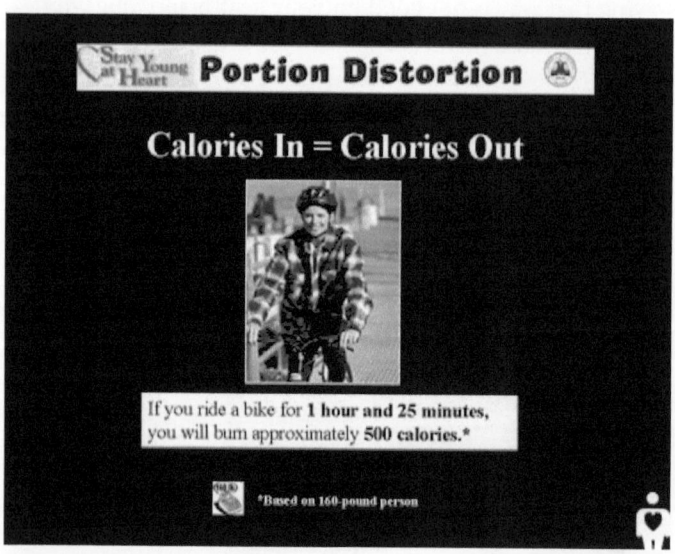

Know your resting **metabolic rate** (RMR), it represents the number of calories you are burning while being totally inactive. Your basal metabolic rate (BMR) is not exactly the same as it is measured after sleeping.

From 60 to 65 percent of calories you eat daily are spent keeping you alive and providing basic energy for life support. While 25 percent of your calories go to movement and physical activity and about 10 percent of calories are spent processing the food you eat.

Thus the formula is simple: to lose weight, you have to reduce calories taken in, increase calories expended, or do both. It is about proportions!

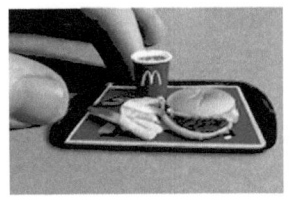

Well, simple? Many overweight people don't burn as many calories as someone of a similar weight with a functional metabolism. We will hand solutions on later pages.

Calculate! Use the appropriate formula for men or women..

Men: BMR = 66 + (13.7 x W) + (5 x H) - (6.8 x Age) = Daily calories required

Women: BMR = 665 + (9.6 x W) + (1.8 x H) - (4.7 x Age) = Daily calories needs

Where: W = weight in Kgs ; H = Height in cms (1 foot = 12 inches, 1 inch = 2.54 cms) and Age = Years

An example for a 30 year old women weighing 80 (176 pounds) Kgs and 5 foot 6 inches tall would be:

665 + (9.6 x 80) + (1.8 x 168) - (4.7 x 30) thus **1590 calories** per day! For a man with the same parameters it would be +200 calories more (1796 cal). If the woman's weight was 130 pounds (59 kg) her BMR would be only 1390 calorie.

Multiply your BMR by an activity factor which more closely suits your lifestyle to find your **true daily caloric needs**.
Your **metabolic rate** = your **resting metabolic rate** + **energy consumed** by your daily activities.

Sedentary - none or very little exercise, desk job = BMR X 1.2
!!Most of us are in this situation!!
Light activity for average of 2 days/week = BMR X 1.375
Moderate activity level exercising 4 days/week = BMR X 1.5
High activity levels exercise & sports more than 6 days/week = BMR X 1.7
Higher activity levels, physical job = up to 2 x BMR

Your RMR and BMR will go down with aging, less height and less weight.
While getting older you should then eat less and/or exercise more.
If you have a 'low' metabolism and thus a lower RMR than average you will burn

less calories at rest and you will gain faster weight than people with a 'high' metabolism.

Be accountable for calories. You need a general idea of how many calories you need. An average **woman**, not an athlete, in her 40s or 50s, needs about **2000 calories** a day, on average, if she is exercising.
A middle-aged **man**, average height and not an athlete but exercising, needs about **2600 calories**.

Your metabolism or 'metabolic rate': the higher it is the more calories (present in your food and drinks) you burn and the more energy is released.

You are normal: most people are very confused about nutrition and calories. If you are not familiar with calorie charts than don't start using them. Keep it simple. Use your common sense and our many balancing "**EnjoyVity**" advices.

So to **slim down or balance your weight** you should

1) Get **less** calories per day IN than you need
2) Increase your RMR and metabolism. In general, the more muscle we have, the higher our metabolic rate; the less muscle we have, the lower our metabolic rate.
   A person's metabolism burns on average 70% of all daily calories - the remainder is burned through physical activity. So the main problem in people who are overweight is their body's failure to burn calories efficiently through metabolism.

Metabolism: metabolism is the rate at which your body burns calories. 'Thermogenesis' is the process of heat production thus energy burning. The measure of metabolism is the quantity of energy released by time unit and by m^2 of skin expressed in J/m^2 or W/m^2, while a **MET** = 58 W/m^2 for a relaxing/sitting person. Compare:

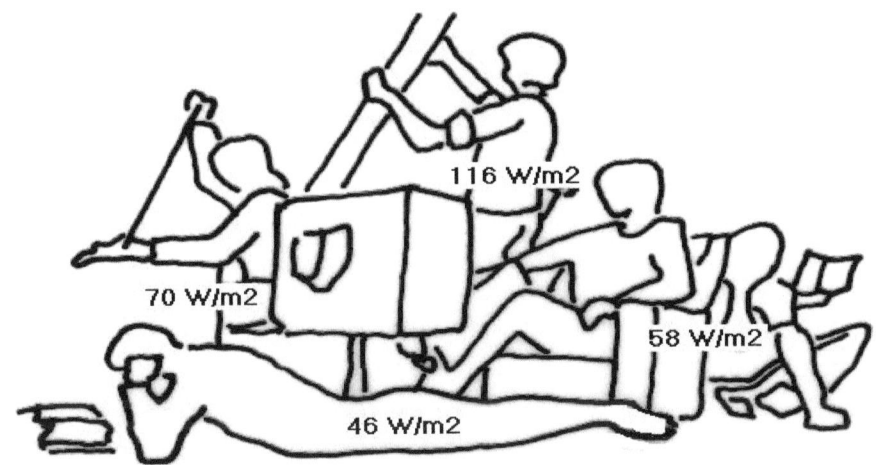

Understand: with a daily energy intake of **1500 kcal** per day still gain weight means you have a **LOW metabolism** and if your daily intake is **3500 kcal** and you still loose weight then you have a **HIGH** metabolism and/or you are in 'top-sports'.

Our body and brain is unaware of our Western Food Security and makes fat layers as energy reserves for possible periods of winter colds and food shortage. **Boosting of your metabolism** will release energy and increase fat burning and the excretion of fluids. This is the way to mislead your intelligent built-in survival instinct which makes you craving for food.

Why your metabolism can be LOW:

- Fasting or serious abrupt calorie-reduction can dramatically reduce BMR by up to 30%
- A overall restrictive low calorie diet can make BMR drop also till 20%
- Snacking high sugared foods throughout the day (candy, colas, cakes, gum).
- Eating or drinking too much sugar containing foods.
- Lack of physical activity.
- Under active thyroid.
- Genetics
- Gender: woman have lower BMR
- Age: BMR reduces with age (~2%/decade)
- Weight: thin women have 25% lower BMR compared to obese women
- Body Fat Percentage: the higher your body fat percentage, the lower your BMR
- Body Temperature: the slower the metabolic rate the lower the normal body temperature

12+3 metabolism boosters:

1. Build muscles, as they need more energy than fat to maintain itself (workout with music)
2. Sport more often as it increases your muscle mass; from brisk walking till rope jumping to get your heart beat up; 20'x5/week
3. Moving even incidental in day-to-day activities increases your thermo-genesis (energy burning); jeans wearers with comfortable shoes walk ~490 steps more a day; squeezing your butt while walking burns (not only) extra calories
4. Lower your surroundings-/room temperature (*). Take a sauna or IR bath it speeds up your blood circulation and overall improves your metabolism, but combine with or separately take morning cold shower or chill out for extra metabolism stimulation
5. Drink enough water as dehydrating lowers your metabolism (your water need=your water desire + 1/3). 1 liter/30kg or 60 pounds of weight; add spoon of apple cider vinegar/lt.
6. Drink 'green' tea daily it has many beneficial effects and also improves the fat burning
7. Avoid alcohol, sugar, and fastings
8. Eat +100 gram of proteins per day; choose among lean meat, skinless chicken, oily fish and low-fat dairy products; yoghourt
9. Use spices and especially hot pepper (chili) and horseradish it stimulates your heartbeat
10. Eat more but smaller healthy portions (3 meals + 3 healthy in between snacks) a day; cut out fried foods, limit salt and sugars and go for high-fiber vegetables and cereals, fruits and proteins; always have breakfast and keep your dinner light and 4 hours before bedtime. Add fibers to foods wherever you can, it are 'superboosters'.
11. Watercress stimulates metabolism and digestion and will reduce oxidative stress; mix with balsamic, olive oil and onion or garlic for a fresh low calorie salad
12. Avoid emotional and physical stress
13. Sleep enough (minimum 6.5 hours) but not too much (maximum 9 hours)
14. Eat natural foods (non-processed) which your body will metabolize correctly
15. Get a thorough body massage, it not only increases metabolism but heals, relaxes and refreshes the muscles and improves detox

(*)The colder the temperature, the more people tend to eat, which is why restaurants often keep thermostats (very) low. "Your metabolism drops when it's time to eat, and eating warms you up," says David Ludwig, professor of pediatrics at Harvard.

Start to check with your practitioner before engaging in sport, extreme exercises or starting any herbs or supplements; overweight can also be due to an underactive thyroid.

Important: be patient with yourself. It took years to create these habits. It is going to take some time to replace them with good ones. Go gradual while you change your old habits to your new ones. This way the change will have a better chance of actually sticking. Meaning that you don't change in a day from drinking 4 glasses of your favorite milk or Coke to 4 glasses of pure water, but you change every other day by one glass. The same for the other unhealthy drinking or eating habits you may have. Change step by step fried foods for steamed vegetables, white bread for full grain passing over half-full wheat bread or processed foods for fresh whole foods.

Anyhow we are **not talking diet** here. "**EnjoyVity**" is not about being hungry or not be able to enjoy your meals, well to the contrary as you will learn.

Eating healthy is not the same as being a 'healthfood junky'. Don't be too strict on food, don't become afraid to eat, your 'diet' should not make you socially isolated. Steven Bratman, M.D., called '**orthorexia**' when healthy eating becomes an obsession. So it is a true eating disorder, like anorexia nervosa or bulimia and needs treatment with professional help.

Low calorie eating habits: don't make it end up as another diet which forces you to calculate calories and feel frustrated. Eating well does not mean eat low or less. Nevertheless, what is wrong in having a slight hunger feeling? It makes you alert, desire, dream and it sure feels better than an upset stomach.

Calorie restriction! Has shown to "decelerate aging" in mice and rhesus monkeys; when those animals were fed 30% to 40% fewer calories they live 30% to 40% longer. No matter how well CR works in people, the maniacal stoicism it demands from 'CRONies' (Calorie Restriction with Optimal Nutrition) will be too much for most. How many of us are willing to eat like birds for the rest of our lives—and to endure the bony frames, constant chill, and lowered libido that frequently accompany a CR regime?

According to recent scientists studies at Washington University School of Medicine in St. Louis however, the Calorie restriction diet that is low in calories and high in nutrition, may not be as effective at extending life in people as it is in rodents.

And! A nutrition researcher in San Diego suspected that the life-extending effects of calorie restriction might be the result of a decreased intake of toxins. He removed the toxic heavy metals from foods, and found that the animals which ate a **normal amount** of food lived as long as the semi-starved animals. Recently, the iron content of food has been identified as the major life-shortening factor, rather than the calories. [Choi and Yu, Age vol. 17, page 93, 1994.]

While you change your eating habits like described in this chapter your body will or might let you know by headaches, bloating, and nausea. It means that your body is throwing out toxics and has begun to cleanse and adapt to a healthier new you! Continue as it is only temporarily and it also does not mean that these whole foods are bad for you, ok.

See weight loss as a by-product of 'healthy' eating and focus on improving your nutritional intake.

The right **supplements** for you, OK, but a daily OVERDOSE of vitamins, antioxidants, probiotics, ... do NOT compensate for unhealthy eating and living habits. An FDA survey shows that about 40 percent of the general population takes supplements daily, with women taking more than men. Among the elderly, surveys show that between 66 and 72 percent take supplements. It's also estimated that 5 to 10 percent of the people who take supplements ingest 'mega-doses', defined by some researchers as ten times the USRDA or more, of certain vitamins and minerals.

Supplements are exactly that, to supplement a normal balanced diet and need to be taken in moderation and not over long periods of time. Even at lower dosages, always monitor yourself carefully and respect the feedback your body provides. Remember in many studies even a placebo vial will help.

By the way also a **NO** to **Human Growth Hormones (HGH)! Still, the drug is at the center of a growing medical and legal controversy.** Anyhow decreased HGH in our body, like during a starvation period, is in recent studies linked to lengthening our life span. Further was found that performance rose even when athletes mistakenly thought they were taking growth hormone, researchers say.

Get informed: 'hghwatch.com' and know that before making decisions that impact upon your health, you should consult your health care provider. **Whole food first**, then in function of your age a Vitamin and supplement program tailored to your individual needs can help you to overcome shortness.

Choose then always for a quality and reliable source.

Listen to your body: become conscious of the reasons for wanting to eat, whether it is true hunger for energy which you hope to find in food or eating for other reasons such as stress, worries, troubles, loneliness, or depression.

Psychological help may be needed to make you understand better your behavior and show ways to improve your social or family relationships and build your self-image and esteem.

If you have a chronicle eating disorder like anorexia, bulimia or compulsive overeating you should consult a healthcare professional to start with.

Understand about your body's **Biorhythm** and its three daily periods: 1) from 12 till 8 PM (20.00) eating and digestion 2) from 8 PM till 4 AM (04.00) assimilation and absorption and 3) between 4 AM and 12 AM (noon) elimination of body waste and remainders of food.

Variety is **KEY**. Buy and eat different colored fruit and vegetables grown on organic farms. Note that just 70 years ago there were no other than organic farms and there was no overweight and obesity epidemic.

Learn from the past: Grain products and concentrated sugars were essentially absent from human nutrition until the invention of agriculture, which was only 10,000 years ago. Animals and humans in traditional tribal societies manage to stay slim without dieting or gym memberships.

By 1980 western foods such as white bread, **refined sugar,** jam, canned and processed foods as well as tobacco and alcohol had become popular in most outskirts of the world and with them their associated diseases.

Right now there is no proven **magic pill** to keep you fit and extend your life. Step away from malnutrition. Food is intended to feed your body with energy. If you eat empty foods you are fooling yourself. Eat healthy and balanced.

Move. Think Positive. Believe.

What is then right to eat:

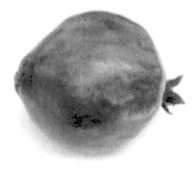

Humans are **omnivores** and need animal protein as well as plant foods to maintain sound health.

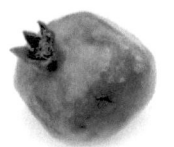

Pomegranate: a powerful antioxidant drink, and can be very important for your health, and has around 3 times more antioxidants than red wine, green tea and cranberry juice, contains also all the important minerals and vitamins required by our body. Use as fresh fruit or as juice. If you drink one glass of pomegranate juice a day, you may be able to reduce high blood pressure and LDL cholesterol (the bad cholesterol).

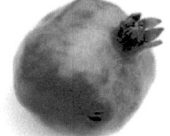

Fermented or pro-biotic the difference: Fermentation breaks down the nutrients in foods by the action of beneficial microorganisms like bacteria and yeast. The end result is foods and drinks that are easier to digest, have more nutrients and are preserved longer. In fact, ancient peoples used this method to preserve foods long before refrigeration! Fermentation is an age-old preparation and preservation technique, increasing your overall nutrition, promoting the growth of friendly intestinal bacteria, and aiding digestion and supporting immune function, including an increase in B vitamins (even Vitamin B12), omega-3 fatty acids, digestive enzymes, lactase and lactic acid, and other immune chemicals that fight off harmful bacteria and even cancer cells. The fermentation was, for Dr. Antoine Bechamp, precursor and opponent of Louis Pasteur, a vital phenomenon of nutrition.

The World Health Organization defines **probiotics** as "live micro-organisms which, when administered in adequate amounts, confer a health benefit". Common strains include Lactobacilli and Bifidobacterium families of bacteria. So it is all about 'friendly' bacteria. Note that there are more bacteria in just one person's intestines than there are human beings in the world.

Prebiotics are non-digestible foods that make their way through our digestive system and help good bacteria grow and flourish, they mostly come from carbohydrate **fibers** called oligosaccharides, as in fruit, whole grains and legumes.

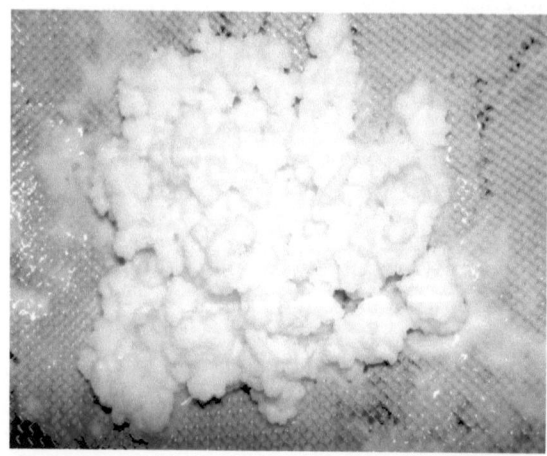

Kefir flowers or grains needed to start the fermentation process.

Kefir is a specific fermented milk product and as such also a pro-biotic it contains beneficial yeast as well as the friendly 'probiotic' bacteria found in yoghurt; it is around, especially in Eastern Europe and Central Asia, for centuries, probably millennia. The health benefits of this traditionally lacto-fermented food are multiple. It contributes to a healthy immune system. The process of fermentation adds a

host of beneficial micro-organisms to food, which makes them easier to digest, increasing the healthy flora in our intestinal tracts (beneficial also after the use of antibiotics to restore balance to the digestive tract). You can also make kefir of non milk products like soy-juice; choose a soy milk brand that's made of organically grown full beans and not soy isolates.
Enjoy all the details at Dom's : 'users.sa.chariot.net.au'

Streptococcus thermophilus and *Lactobacillus delbrueckii* spp. *bulgaricus* are the major microbiota in the famous and very tasty Georgian **Matsoni** or fermented milk.

Cultured vegetables are made by shredding cabbage or a combination of cabbage and other vegetables and then packing them tightly into an airtight container. They are left to ferment (without contact with oxygen in a dark environment) at room temperature for several days or longer. Friendly bacteria naturally present in the vegetables quickly lower the pH, making a more acidic environment so the bacteria can reproduce. The vegetables become soft, delicious, and somewhat "pickled", as example sauerkraut. The Chinese have been fermenting cabbage for thousands of years. Learn more about fermentation: 'wildfermentation.com'

Fibers and complete not refined flour! Add bulk fibers as '**wheat bran**' to your preparations like salads, soups, pasta's, … at a rate of **25 gram**/day. Wheat bran is not only a bulking agent, which gives you sooner a satiety feeling, but is rich in minerals, antioxidants, lignans and other phytonutrients-as well as in fiber. They are pr*E*biotics, read above. Fibers normalize your blood sugar levels, help you lose weight, and help prevent colon cancer.
Note that on Greece's countryside there still is a long and strong tradition of all sorts of brown breads, including a fermented "shepherd's" loaf made with wheat bran, oat bran and whole wheat flour.

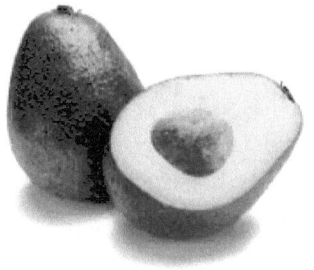

Avocados: are a good source of vitamin K, dietary fiber, vitamin B6, vitamin C, folate, copper and health-promoting monounsaturated fats, especially oleic acid, that may help to lower cholesterol. Avocados are highly enjoyable and creamy. Use them as bread spread, in your salads, dressings and as a garnish wherever possible.

Horseradish contains more than 10-fold higher glucosinolates, compounds that has been shown to increase human resistance to cancer, than broccoli. Support your body's production of "good" estrogens while decreasing the "bad" ones and stimulate the detoxification systems of the 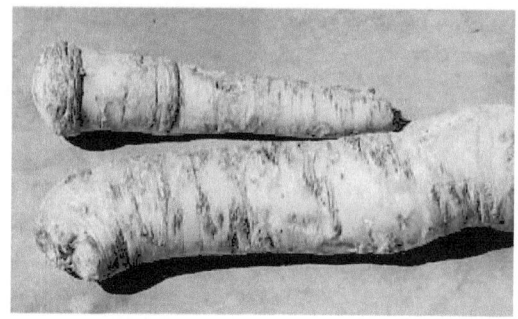 body. Known as an aphrodisiac, a treatment for rheumatism . Japanese horseradish is also called wasabi. One teaspoon a day! See also our 'garladior'. The consumption of horseradish is not advisable to individuals suffering from gastric ulcer, goitrous problems or renal illnesses.

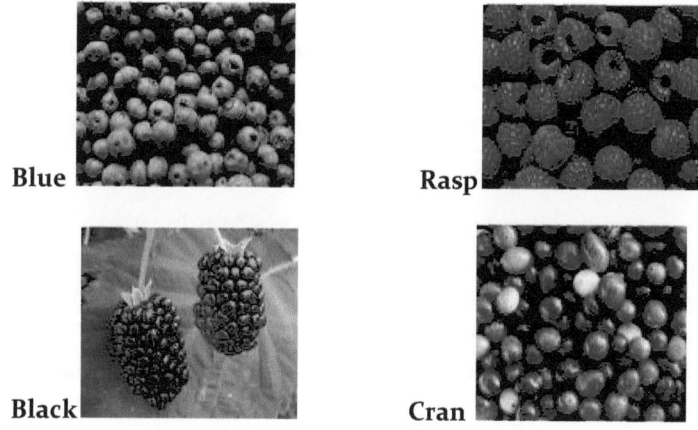

Blue Rasp

Black Cran

Blueberries are a very powerful fruit to eat. This is definitely the kind of fruit you would want to include in your anti aging regimen. Adding Blueberries will help cleanse your blood, strengthen your immune system, great for your digestion, and even help keep colds at bay, and don't forget you are protecting and repairing your skin.

Raspberries: Raspberries are in the top 10 high antioxidant fruits and vegetables. Rich in vitamin C, folate, iron and potassium, raspberries also provide high amounts of insoluble fiber (thanks to all those little seeds) as well as respectable amounts of the soluble fiber pectin, which helps control cholesterol levels.

Blackberries rank highly among fruits for antioxidant strength, particularly due to their dense contents of polyphenolic compounds,tannins,, ellagitannins, quercitin, gallic acid, anthocyanins and cyanidins. They are in the **TOP 10** on the ORAC list; **Oxygen Radical Absorbance Capacity** (ORAC) is a method of measuring antioxidant capacities of different foods. Look at page 73 for the USDA data on

foods with high levels of antioxidant phytochemicals.
Cranberries are rich in antioxidants and play a role in maintaining cardiovascular health and were shown to decrease total cholesterol and LDL or "bad" cholesterol levels in a recent study conducted by the University of Wisconsin-Madison. Amy Howell, Ph.D., of Rutgers University: "Cranberries contain compounds that have an anti-adhesion or anti-stick mechanism that's been shown to be effective in maintenance of urinary tract health".

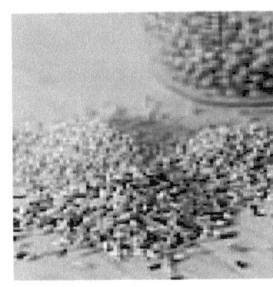

Buckwheat: is not a wheat for starters; a 'whole grain' yes it is actually **a fruit seed** that is related to rhubarb and sorrel making it a suitable substitute for grains for people who are sensitive to wheat or other grains that contain protein **gluten**s. A tasteful basic and great alternative for rice, potatoes, pasta's, ... ready in minutes and universally usable in your kitchen. A perfect food, ideally nutritive and dynamic, it is completely assimilable being itself organic and alive.

Why? The grain has an amino acid composition nutritionally superior to all cereals, including oats. Buckwheat contains linoleic acid, vitamins (B1, B2, B3, B5, E, P), essential amino acids, minerals - chromium, copper, manganese, folic acid - and is an excellent source of magnesium. It has anti-tumor and tonic effects. Due to the presence of inosit, buckwheat adjusts metabolism, fat and the lipo-soluble vitamins. It also helps the liver in processing hormones, medicines, and glucoses, with a protective hepatic effect. Buckwheat provides the necessary amount of proteins necessary for the body because it contains essential amino acids which the body cannot synthesize and who need to be taken from one's daily nutrition. Buckwheat decreases the cholesterol level by eliminating fat and assuring protection against arthrosclerosis. It prevents the developing of biliary lithiasis by optimizing the synthesizing of biliary acids and eliminating neutral and acid fat. Owing to the quantity of magnesium contained, buckwheat has a relaxing effect over blood vessels, improving circulation and decreasing blood pressure. Because it contains plenty of vitamins with B complex, buckwheat is recommended in cases of liver disorders and sugary diabetes, illnesses where it is unadvisable to increase the quantity of sugary substances consumed each day. Due to the fact that it lacks sugary substances makes buckwheat ideal for those who need to keep a restrictive diet. This herb offers protection against breast cancer as well as against other forms of cancer dependent on hormones. Through the contained antioxidants buckwheat is an antidote for X-ray irradiations or other forms of irradiation. Read more at 'whfoods.com'

Flax Seed – a must have in your diet, both ground meal and whole. The oil in the flax "greases" up your arteries and cleans them out so to speak as well as cleaning out your bowels. Dump flax into anything you can. Hide it in spaghetti, yogurt, stir fry, anything because once this seed actually elevated your HDL which is your good cholesterol and gives you a preventative measure. Flaxseed is easily ground in a coffee grinder, food processor, or blender, and may be added to foods such as hot cereals, salads, or smoothies.

Garlic: as fresh garlic cloves, its juice, dried powder for kitchen use or in oral capsules (*) never enough - step up your garlic consumption. Not only is it good for your heart but it is a natural anti-coagulant so it thins the blood and prevents clotting and it has the equivalent of antibiotic properties. Good preventative measures for heart attack and stroke. Garlic is a great source of non-digestible **'inulin'**. This allows it to pass through the small intestine and ferment in the large intestine. Through the fermentation process, the inulin becomes healthy intestinal microflora (bifido-bacterium). Read also on healthy fibers and inuline at 'prebiotic.ca' .

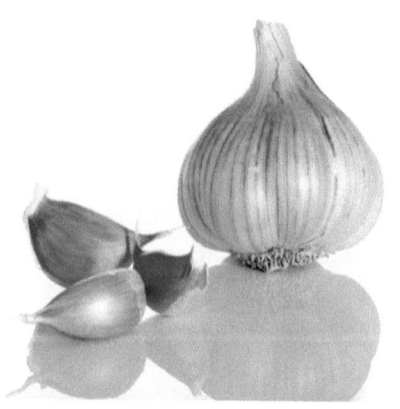

If you love garlic, eat it raw or use its freshly pressed juice all-over, or roast an entire bulb in the oven for 40 minutes and squeeze it out onto a piece of toasted whole bread once a day. You hate garlic! Why? Think again, it is about 'Your' health.

- Natural antibiotic and antiviral agent as a result of sulfur-containing compounds
- May help with infections: colds, sore throat, ear infections in children, fungal or yeast infections
- May slow development of atherosclerosis, improve high blood pressure and decrease total and LDL (bad) cholesterol by reducing blood platelet stickiness and artery spasms
- May decrease risk of developing colorectal, prostate, breast, liver, skin, and digestive tract cancers by inhibiting the growth of tumors and stimulating the immune system

You can cover the garlic breath by chewing some fresh parsley during use and the next day when important meetings are up. You can also cut out the germ sprout in

the middle of the clove, it will help greatly against garlic breath. There are too many health benefits linked to garlic that you would consider, due to the breath issue, for not using it almost daily. Best is to convince friends or relatives also to become 'garlicophiles'!
Put in your FAQ while looking for a partner : Smoking NO, garlic YES.
You must factor this into your diet somehow, someway.
(*) odor free garlic capsules are on the market, so no further excuse.

Ginger : a spice which is used for cooking and is also consumed whole as a delicacy or medicine. Health care professionals commonly recommend it to help prevent or treat nausea and vomiting associated with motion sickness, pregnancy, and cancer chemotherapy. It is also used as a digestive aid for mild stomach upset, as support in inflammatory conditions such as arthritis, and may even be used in heart disease or cancer. Indeed does its outspoken 'BEV' parameters and a very negative PRAL (*) show that the fresh juice has definite 'terrain' corrective properties. (*) a negative PRAL figure shows the alkalizing effect of the 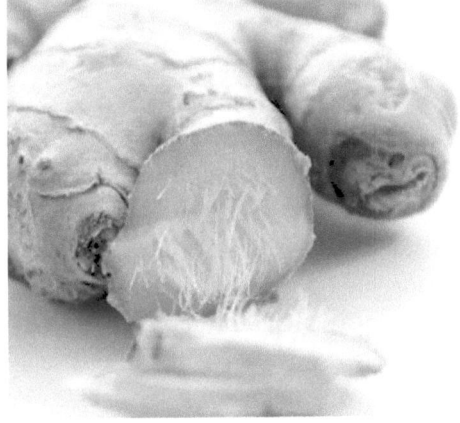 food on the body and a positive figure its acidifying properties. Read somewhat further on your **acid/alkaline balance** and the **BEV-terrain** chapter 6.

Seaweed healthy food: wild sea greens can help to build and sustain the broad nutritional balance of vitamins, minerals and vital nutrients on which optimum health and vitality depend. The use of depleted soil/pesticide and herbicides (modern farming) and food processing worsens this imbalance in our common foods.

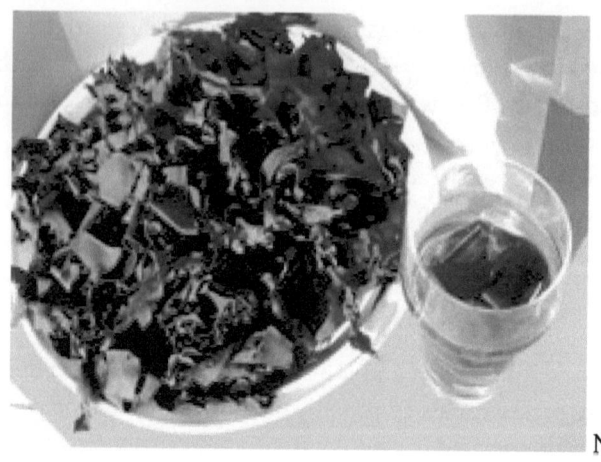
Nori or wakame seaweed

It has been estimated that certain seaweeds are up to 30 times higher in minerals than land food, which is affected by depleted nutrient levels in our soils. Modern diet tends to favor carbohydrates, protein and fats, which can all become surplus **acid deposits** if our bodies do not have the means to fully metabolize them. Seaweed can neutralize these acids so they can be safely eliminated and help restore balance. Seaweed is a good source of selenium, magnesium, potassium, iron, iodine and trace elements. It has anti-cancer effects while providing soluble fibers and omega 3 fats. It promotes thyroid health. Sea greens, come in different colors and are a perfect source of proteins (up to 45%), carbs as soluble fibers, insoluble fibers, phyto-chemicals, essential fatty acids and anti-oxidants. Seaweed and algae contain small amounts of all of the essential glycol-nutrients which you do need for your body to function properly. They are at the basis of communication between cells, delivering the messages that enable cells to work together to keep your body healthy and balanced.
More details: '**wildseagreens.com**' or 'seaweedireland.com'.

Some of our favorite recipes:

'**Bucky**', salad for 2 persons: 150 gram of buckwheat grains, cook as rice in pure water, add one raw grated carrot, one fresh cucumber diced in small cubes, a cup of yoghourt, soupspoon of olive oil, dash of soya sauce, fresh coriander leaves or your favorite green herbs. Mix and enjoy!

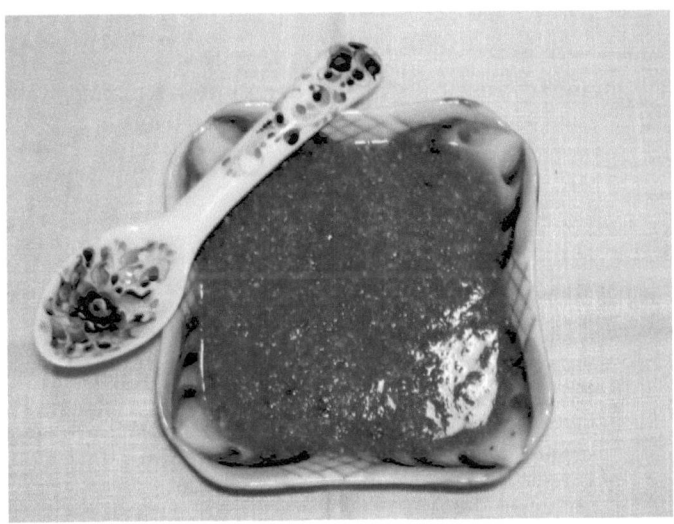

'**Garladior**': your cocktail of life or your full Mendeleev mineral table. Clean a fresh horseradish beet (~300 gram) and cut it in your kitchen blender, add one or two fresh cleaned garlic bulb(s), as well as 2 pounds (1kilo) of tomatoes, one sweet red paprika and 300 gram of apple, nice spoon of sea-salt mix it all together put it in closed jars in fridge and enjoy from next day on.

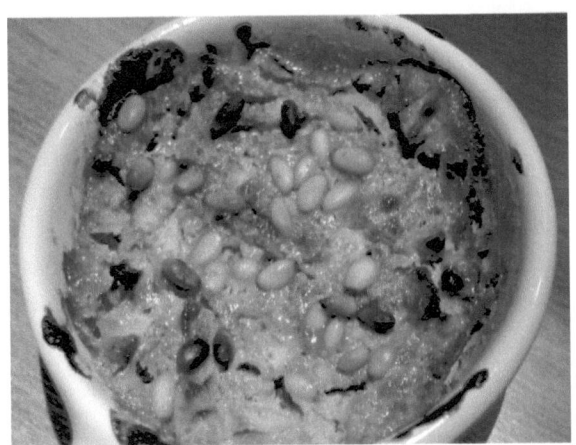

'**Happy Soul' cake:** mash 200 gram cottage cheese in blender then add and mix with 2 eggs, 2 spspoon of bran, 3 spspoon brown sugar add to it all enough pre-diced fresh or sundried apricots. Oil a baking form and cover with bran-fibers and throw on your 'Soul' mixture. Bake it in oven for 30' at 360F/180C. Enjoy warm or cold. Be happy.

'**Nufu**': our nuts-cheese salad mixture. Add to iceberg or rocket salad leaves, portions cubes of fresh goat cheese (75 gram/person)(make it yoghourt or curd if goat cheese is not your favorite), add your favorite almonds or nuts, sunflower seeds, pumpkin seeds, fresh or sundried red grapes and mix with ½ cup of Bifidus yoghourt, soya sauce, honey, apple vinegar and spsp olive oil.

'**Minus**'-**snack** with mixed nuts and seeds: use equal amounts of flax seeds, sunflower seeds, pumpkin seeds, dry apricot and prunes, almonds, walnuts, macadamia-nuts or pistachios and pine kernels; a true heart protection.

"**EnjoyVity**" **flour:** ground together these quantities buckwheat (1) (*), sesam (1/2), whole oat flakes (1), pine kernel (1/2), flax seed (1/2), wheat-bran(1/2) and unrefined seasalt (1/8). (*) 1 soup spoon equals 2 persons serving

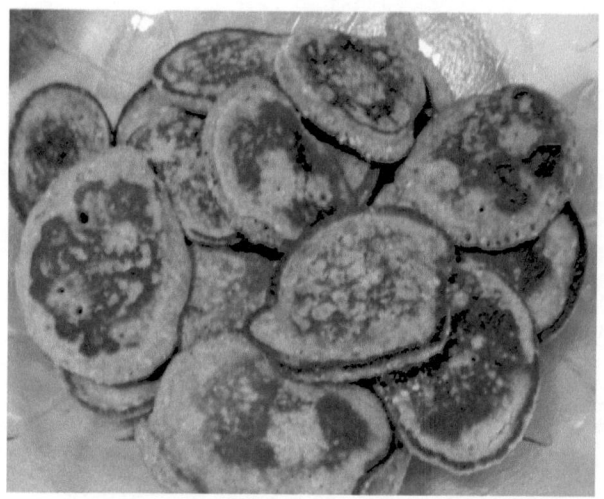

With this flour you make:
a) '**EnjoyVital**'-**porridge:** add lukewarm water or milk or soya-juice to the desired quantity of the 'EnjoyVity' flour mix, stir wait 5 minutes and enjoy with your favorite seasonal fruit, honey, maple syrup, ...

b) '**EnjoyVital**'-**fritters:** add 1 or 2 raw scrambled eggs, pancake flour (2) and a dash of water or milk, stir and bake in oil as usual
c) '**EnjoyVital**'-**fooDballs**: add a fresh scrambled egg to desired volume of 'EV'flour and roll them into small balls which. Great for soup or to bake in oil as such.

'**VITY**-salad': for 2 persons in a large salad bowl toss together 100 gram rucola (rocket) salad, one avocado in dices, 125 gram river-crayfish, Spspn pinenuts (slightly roasted), five fresh or sundried prunes cut in slices, small sweet red onion, 2 Spspn of salsa paprika, flavor with liquid mountain honey, virgin olive oil, curcuma, red pepper, soy sauce and finish with a dash of truffle oil. Enjoy slowly 'without' bread.

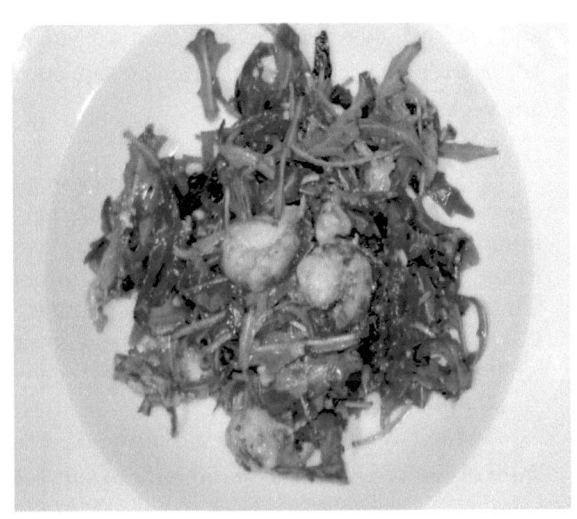

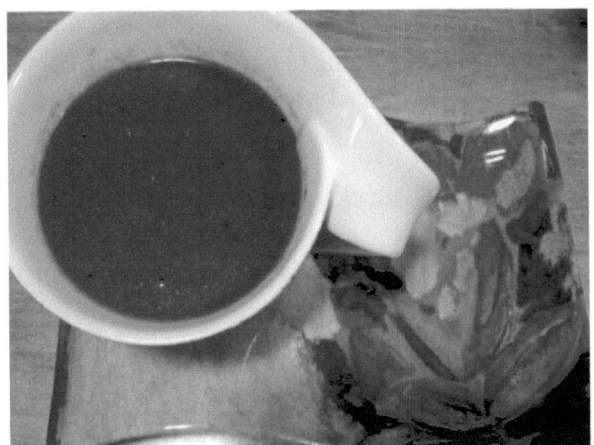

'**Chosou**' **soup:** chop one onion and carrot add to 0.5 liter of hot water, seasalt or seaweed mixture, a chunk of ginger, add 250 gr of brown sliced fungi and cook 3'; mix in blender and finish with 20 gram of fibers; put back on stove to melt and add 8 gr of +80% black **chocolate**. Stir and taste.

"EnjoyVital" -dip: crush with hand-mixer 300 gram fresh green grapes and 300 gram blackberries; squeeze out and recuperate the juice with a sieve or prepare in juice-maker; warm the juice and cool down; ground 250 gram walnuts add the the juice of 4 garlic-cloves, 2 precut twigs of coriander and some sea salt; add the fruit-juice to the walnut mixture; you can keep it for 2 weeks in fridge but better to enjoy with steamed fish, chicken, cucumber salad, brown pasta or with any vegetable.

'Space Syrup' elixir: 2 tsp. diced fresh garlic, 3 Tbs. olive oil, 5 Tbs. pure clover honey, 1 Tbs. apple cider vinegar, 1/2 tsp. cayenne, 1/4 tsp. 'asafoetida' (optional, has calming effect on central nervous system), 1/4 cup strong green tea, freshly made. Sauté garlic in olive oil for 1 minute, then add other ingredients. Simmer and cook over low flame for 5 minutes. Let cool. Strain into glass jar. Cover and refrigerate. Use one teaspoon a day and evaluate yourself after a month what the elixir brought for you; recipe as received by Mrs. Ritkiss/CA

Healthy spread: Let virgin olive oil partially solidify in the fridge. Add a snuff of sea-salt and fresh garlic-juice to suit your taste and put it back in fridge to solidify.

You are going to **cook more yourself** in order to keep control of your own health. If being less experienced you get confused about measurements look here for the right spoon, gram, cup or ounce 'envoyvity.com/measurement-equivalents' or at the table in the back of the book.

Although not always practical for working-outside-families it would be best for your bodies digestion, assimilation and calorie burning to have a good breakfast and lunch while your dinner will be light and finished 3 hours before going vertical/to sleep.

No Time! Try 'Fast' : indeed fasting is from all times and from all religions; try practicing 24 hours fasting once a   month or even several days in a row at start of spring season and autumn; combine with a soft herbal detoxification program for blood, liver, bowel and kidney.

Say **YES** to the **Slow Food** movement, which promotes regionally grown goods and local culinary traditions. A new hype? Yes, but think it over ... organic, local, and seasonal! And definitely much more balanced, healthy and vital than those of the 'quick food'-culture. Great! Team up, for a better, healthier and sustainable world: 'slowfood.com' .

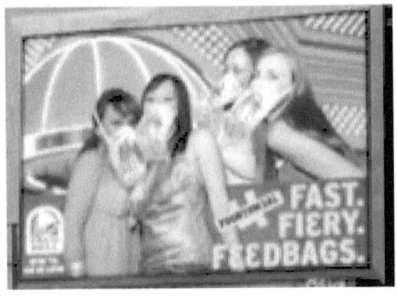

Say **NONONO** to the **wearable Feedbag**. Just look, no further comments!

'naturalnews.com'

Fresh produce and olive oil can't always compete with hamburgers and fries. We, spoiled humans, are attracted to, but not designed to handle the fast food diet. **The desire for food sensation has obviously gone far beyond the needs of the body. ~Karl Loren**
That is why the 'Mediterranean diet' is dying out even in Greece, Italy or Spain. And why in Greece, three-quarters (!) of the adult population is now overweight or obese.

The '**Mediterranean diet**', from populations bordering the Mediterranean Sea, has (*we should thus better use 'had'*) the reputation for being a model of healthy eating and contributing to better health and quality of life. **It is rich in olive oil, grains, fruits, nuts, honey, vegetables, and fish, but low in meat, dairy products and alcohol.** And it came about without advice of universities, State associations, doctors, food industry, ...

The 'old style' **Okinawans** eat on average 500 calories less per day than other social groups however the diet is not simply about calorie restriction but also emphasizes the selection of highly nutritious foods. The recommended foods are low in calories but high in flavor and nutrients. See also chapter 11 and 'okinawaprogram.com'.

For all and the **too many type of diets** look 'later' at everydiet.org and then still start with 'karlloren.com'.

Antioxidants: Measure where you stand with the instant and n**on-invasive Raman Spectroscopy or** Biophotonic scanner. Your Skin Carotenoid Score is an immediate numeric reading of your own skin carotenoid content and an important indicator of the overall strength of your body's antioxidant defense system. It will give you an indication how your body is aging.
See 'pharmanexscanner.com'

> **"The amount of key antioxidants that many different species maintain in their body is directly proportional to their lifespan"**
> ~ Dr. Richard Cutler, M.D., Director of Anti-aging research at the US National Institute of Health.

Keep those **antioxidant** levels high: When we eat plants that have large amounts of antioxidants, our bodies can use those same substances to repair damage to our own cells, caused by the "free radicals". There are many different health conditions that antioxidants can help to prevent, including heart disease, macular degeneration, diabetes, cancer, and liver disease. Substances research believes inhibit cancer include vitamin C, vitamin E, beta-carotene, selenium, and gluthione (related to amino acid). These substances are all reducing agents. They supply electrons to free radicals and block the interaction of the free radical with normal tissue.

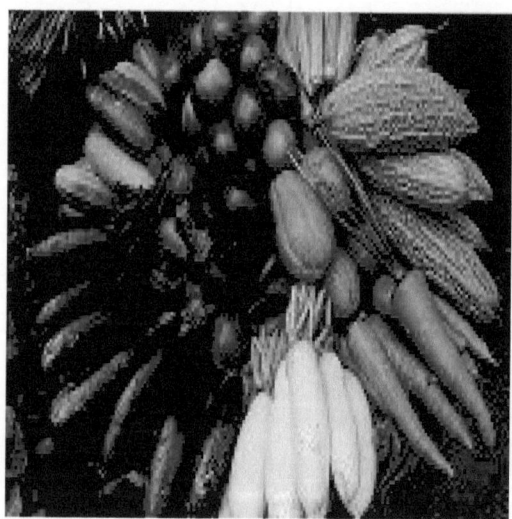

Fruits, vegetables, legumes and herbs with the darkest colors contain most of them. Some examples are dark berries, dark red kidney beans and dark skinned potatoes, carrots, squash, broccoli, sweet potatoes, tomatoes, kale, cabbage, Brussels sprouts, collards, spinach, apricots, and all bright colored fruits (like mango, papaya) and vegetables are high in antioxidants. Flax- seed, oatmeal, barley, rye, grapefruit, watermelon, and tea are all high in antioxidants as well. Many protein-rich foods such as chicken, shellfish, fish and red meats also contain antioxidants. The 'top' is found in black chocolate! But again use with moderation and step by step as over doing it harms.

Antioxidant Levels of Common Foods; source U.S. Department of Agriculture

FOOD	PORTION	ANTIOXIDANT LEVEL
dried red beans	1/2 cup	13727
wild blueberries	1 cup	13427
dried red kidney bean	1/2 cup	13259
pinto beans	1/2 cup	11864
Blueberries	1 cup	9019
whole cranberries	1 cup	8983
cooked artichoke hearts	1 cup	7904
Blackberries	1 cup	7701
Prunes	1/2 cup	7291
Raspberries	1 cup	6085
Strawberries	1 cup	5938
red delicious apples	1 apple	5900
granny smith apples	1 apple	5381
Pecans	1 ounce	5095
sweet cherries	1 cup	4873
black plum	1	4844
cooked Russet potato	1	4649
dried black beans	1/2 cup	4181
Plum	1	4118

Missing in this 'ORAC' table is **red beet** though it is unique for its high levels of anti-carcinogens and its very high carotenoid content.
It sure ends up number 1 on my list.
Betacyanin is the pigment that gives beets their red color; this pigment is absorbed into the blood corpuscles and can increase the oxygen-carrying ability of the blood by up to 400 per cent. Don't throw away the green leafy tops as they can be cooked like spinach and are also rich in beta-carotene, folic acid, chlorophyll, potassium, vitamin C, and iron. When red beets are consumed regularly such as in salad, soups or as beetroot-juice it works as a panacea against diseases.

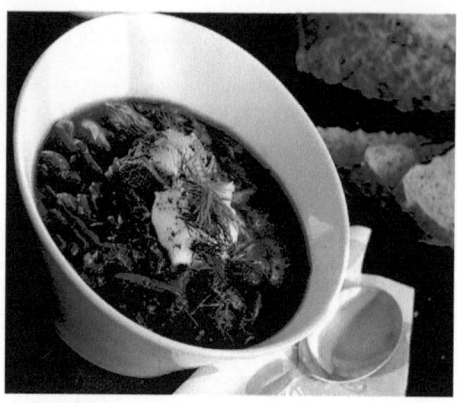
'Borsch'

More for your cardio-vascular health: stay **pro-active**, thus eat as if your life depends on it! To promote cardiovascular health eat mostly vegetables and fruits uncooked, so that their vitamins and fiber are intact. Also meat and fish at best and mostly raw, think sashimi. Know the antioxidant CoenzymQ10 it resembles a fat, behaves like an enzyme, and functions like a vitamin. This supplement will improve heart muscle function while producing no adverse effects, show all mayor studies.

The Reverse List: foods to avoid, try to eliminate all dietary sources of sodium (salt), sodium glutamate, "fast foods", diet soda drinks, baking soda, canned vegetables, commercially prepared packaged foods, foods with preservatives, with added fructose etc.

Soybean products Yes or No: we are over-informed by the soy industry about all the benefic effects of soy products for our health. Mind you, tofu and other soybean foods contain isoflavones, specific molecules bearing a structural resemblance to mammalian steroidal hormones.

One hundred grams of soy protein - the maximum suggested cholesterol-lowering dose can contain almost 600 mg of isoflavones, an amount that is considered undeniably toxic. In 1992, the Swiss health service estimated that 100 grams of soy protein provided the estrogenic equivalent of the Pill.

Another concern: most soy beans are genetically modified, right.
Soybeans are high in phytates, an organic acid that makes it difficult for the body to absorb essential minerals such as calcium, iron, magnesium, and zinc. Phytates are resistant to cooking and can only be reduced by fermentation techniques. Stay thus with **fermented soy** products like tempeh, miso, natto, soy sauce and fermented tofu or milk
Tempeh: This meat substitute is made from soybeans and other grains that have been injected with a mold and allowed to ferment.
Miso: This is a thick paste made from soybeans and grains that has been fermented

and then aged for up to three years. It's a staple in Japan, where it's used to flavor soups, dipping sauces, meats, and dressings.
Natto: Made with fermented soybeans, natto is pungent, sticky, and highly nutritious. The Japanese like to serve it on rice or put it in sushi or miso soups.

Soy products for infants: No! "The amount of phytoestrogens that are in a day's worth of soy infant formula equals 5 birth control pills," says Mary G. Enig, Ph.D., president of the Maryland Nutritionists Association. Many manufacturers do not use the whole soy product in their foods; the protein with the isoflavones is called soy isolates. Soy foods also increase the body's need for vitamin D, and it requires the body to need more vitamin B12.

Myth: Asians consume large amounts of soy foods.
Truth: Average consumption of soy foods in China is 10 grams (about 2 teaspoons) per day and similar amounts in Japan. Asians consume soy foods in small amounts as a condiment, not as a replacement for animal foods and mainly after lengthy fermentation to destroy the soy toxins. Most modern soy foods are not fermented to neutralize toxins in soybeans, and are processed in a way that denatures proteins and increases levels of carcinogens. Read also westonaprice.org

Acid or alkaline foods where is my balance? The ongoing discussion about acidification of our body and the possible sole remedy being re-alkalizing is only part of the truth and even then for many confusing. Just like sour (acid) tasting fruits are alkaline to your body.
Note that when our internal 'tissues' acidify our blood will always be alkalized! When is something acidic then? On the pH scale, which ranges from 0 on the acidic to 14 on the alkaline end, a solution is neutral if its pH is 7. At pH 7, water contains equal concentrations of $H+$ and $OH-$ ions. Substances with a pH less than 7 are acidic because they contain a higher concentration of $H+$ ions. Substances like foods with a pH higher than 7 are alkaline because they contain a higher concentration of $OH-$ than $H+$. When we digest a food it is chemically oxidized ('burned') to form water, carbon dioxide and an inorganic compound. The alkaline or acidic nature of the inorganic compound formed determines whether the food is alkaline or acid-producing. If it contains more sodium, potassium or calcium, it's classed as an alkaline food. If it contains more sulfur, phosphate or chloride, it's classed as an acid food. So a sour thus very acid lemon (pH 2) when digested produces alkaline residue. That's why we classify it as an alkaline food (PRAL-2.5). The pH scale is a logarithmic scale so a change of one pH unit means a tenfold change in the concentration of hydrogen ions. If later we talk about natural spring water with a pH of 6 and an artificial ionized water with a pH of 10 the difference in concentration is a factor 10^4 thus **10.000**! A young and healthy skin has a pH of 5, acid thus.

Importance of balancing pH
Living things are extremely sensitive to pH and function best (with certain exceptions, such as in our stomach) when solutions are nearly neutral. Most 'healthy'

interior living matter has a pH of about 6.8 (**check it out with your urine**).

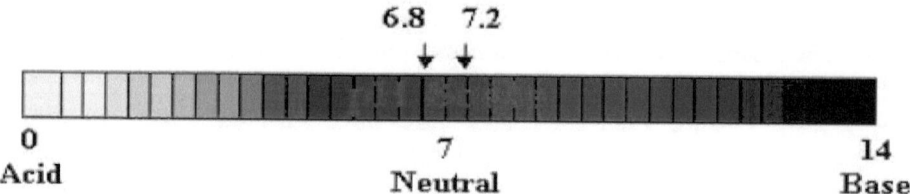

Blood plasma and other fluids that surround the cells in the body have a pH of 7.1 to 7.4. Numerous special mechanisms (buffers) aid in stabilizing these fluids so that cells will not be subject to appreciable fluctuations in pH. **Mesenchyme** is mesodermal tissue that forms connective tissue and blood and smooth muscles. The mesenchym can be acidified, which should be confirmed by measurement first (*), then one best eat only or more food with alkalizing effects in the body in order to shift the 'terrain' (or environment) back again to the neutral pH area.

Venus blood, with an actual (optimal (**)) pH of 7.3-7.35, shifts very rarely towards acidic, but mainly and for all degenerative diseases linked to our modern western lifestyle to alkali (alkalosis). The medical definitions for Acidemia: *blood* pH < 7.36 and *Alkaemia: blood* pH > 7.44 are not identical to the above chemical definitions of acid and alkali pH, which might have lead to more confusion among professionals and patients.

Nevertheless statements as ' the majority of Americans are acidified while having blood pH levels between 6.2-6.4 and need alkaline foods and alkaline water' are absurd, simplifying the medical science and misleading. Let it be known that with a blood pH of 6.2 nobody is still on his feet! Read more page 60 on 'terrain' measurements. Further rH_2 is even more important a measure than pH as a factor in the "Body Electric".

(*)Measure your urine pH (optimal 6.5-6.8) with litmus paper at wake-up and a second time one hour later, if the average score is less than 6 consult your experienced doctor or health practitioner and start an all-round healthy approach of life as explained in this and the next chapters. Same for saliva, with an optimal pH of 6.5-6.75, get advice and sustained correction when you measure sober at wake-up over pH 7.1 (alkali).

(**) Scientists are aware that under our Western lifestyle blood pH is on average shifting more into the alkaline zone. If 50 years ago young people had a blood pH between 7 and 7.1 and today are youngsters score rather between 7.3 and 7.4 it is questionable to define the latter as a healthy blood-pH but rather as one of a pre-degenerative sickness state.

Extra thought: it is measured and known that young healthy disciplined sport athletes still have a blood pH of 7.1.

More food for thought: **Dr. Wilhelm von Brehmer** measured in the 1930-ies blood intra-vascular with his Hämoionometer and noted an average pH of 6,3 at 14 years, 6,8 at 24 years, 7,2 at 40 years, 7,35 at 60 years and 7,6 and over for even older people.

Researches Dr. Remer and Dr. Manz developed a new and more reliable way to measure the acid/base effect of specific foods on the human body. This pH measuring tool is referred to as the Potential Renal Acid Load or **PRAL**. The PRAL factor considers the digestion and absorption of a food and its direct effect on the kidneys and urine. Meats, grains and dairy products, typical parts of a common western diet, are all highly acidic. Vegetables, fruits and nuts are all alkaline. All the foods you have always been told to eat because they are healthy are alkaline forming! Parmesan cheese with a PRAL of 34 is highly acidifying while raisins with a PRAL of -21 are strongly alkalizing. Note that to shift or correct your body substance pH you would need almost to rigorously follow a 'monodiet'. Of course if the current typical Western diet (*) is an acidifying diet it needs correction by adding or better exchanging the grain, meat and dairy products over-consumption by servings of fresh raw vegetables, fruit and nuts; see therefore the logics within this and next chapter. So pH and PRAL values show us clearly that to keep our body substance parameters in optimum balance, which avoid sickness, we need to **eat and drink 'balanced'** and moderately. In PRAL terms eat 2/3 alkalizing and 1/3 acidifying foods. Most of us are eating the other way around or worse, then correction will be needed.

(*) PRAL -39 paleolithic diet (3000Kcal/day) and +23 average US diet today (2500Kcal/day). Reasons for the historical shift from negative to positive PRAL are not only the displacement of alkali-rich plant foods in the ancestral diet by cereal grains and nutrient-poor foods in the temporary diet but also the modern processing and preparation of foods, which lead to considerable losses of base-forming nutrients such as potassium and magnesium.

You can find a table of food and beverages and their PRAL values at 'enjoyvity.com/pral'.

As mentioned while talking about the needed antioxidants in our balanced food the factor next to pH, which is as important and needs consideration, is the content of **FREE ELECTRONS** in and thus the **reducing effect** of our foods. All of us are, more or less, deprived of electrons (*), it is proven that an oxidized interior body environment (at cellular and mithochondrial level) is the underlying fundament for most of our diseases. A balanced healthy menu and lifestyle will bring you these as well alkalizing as reducing elements needed to keep your trillions of cells in optimal condition so they can breathe, get rid of toxics and will not acidify. A good antioxidant will not only bring free electrons, in order to get our body all potentials for the exchange mechanisms, but also consider carefully, without excesses, the protection against the free-radicals. This anti-radical effect of foods is measured with the '**ORAC**', oxygen radical absorbance capacity.

You can find a limited table of food and beverages and their 'ORAC' values page 68 and the BHNRC/USDA based 2007 table at 'enjoyvity.com/orac'

Motivation: a portion of 1,16oz/33 gram of black chocolate will have an ORAC of over 34.000, 0,35oz/10 gram of dried oregano 20.000 and as little as 10 gram of ground cinnamon even 26.700!

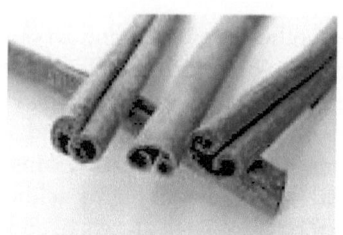

(*) the energy of the electron of the Hydrogen atom is the true fuel of life'~ Albert Szent-Györgyi, Nobel Prize in Physiology, for his discoveries in connection with the biological oxidation/combustion processes, with special reference to vitamin C. He was also one of the first to explore the connections between free radicals and cancer. Disruption of this cellular electron-transfer system by free radicals (highly reactive molecules lacking an electron), Szent-Györgyi suggested, could push cells into the uncontrolled proliferative state that characterizes cancer.

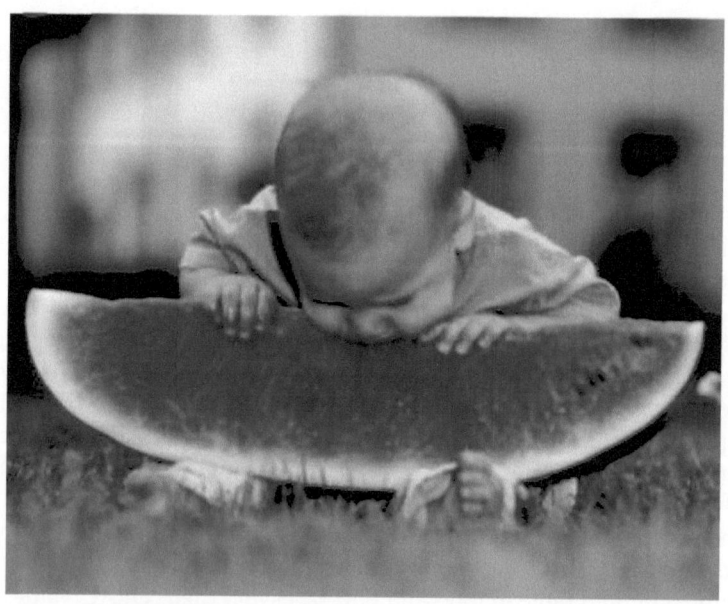

Learn your children to eat healthy!

7 more **"EnjoyVity"** eating advices:

1. Eat less carbohydrates (carbs) strive towards maximum 250 gram /day and even less than 150 gram while controlling your weight. The best sources of carbohydrates—whole grains, vegetables, fruits and beans—promote good health by delivering vitamins, minerals, fiber, and a host of important 'phytonutrients'.
2. Eat more lean protein it will helps in maintaining a high metabolism, helps your immune system and to repair your muscles faster. Take +100 gr/woman or 150 gr/man of lean protein/day. Use therefore lean meats, poultry, fish, beans, eggs, and nuts.
3. Eat plant proteins like beans, soy, consuming 25 grams of "FERMENTED" soy protein daily may also help lower cholesterol and protect against heart disease.
4. Eat 5 to 6 small to medium size meals per day; meaning eat something healthy every 3 hours. This will boost your metabolism. For your main courses you will then eat smaller portions.
5. Don't finish a meal hungry but stop 'as soon' you feel satisfied.
6. Be conscious of what you eat but without having to be ascetic.
7. Delicious, attractive, fresh, and minimally cooked (better raw or steamed) whole foods are the great way to go.

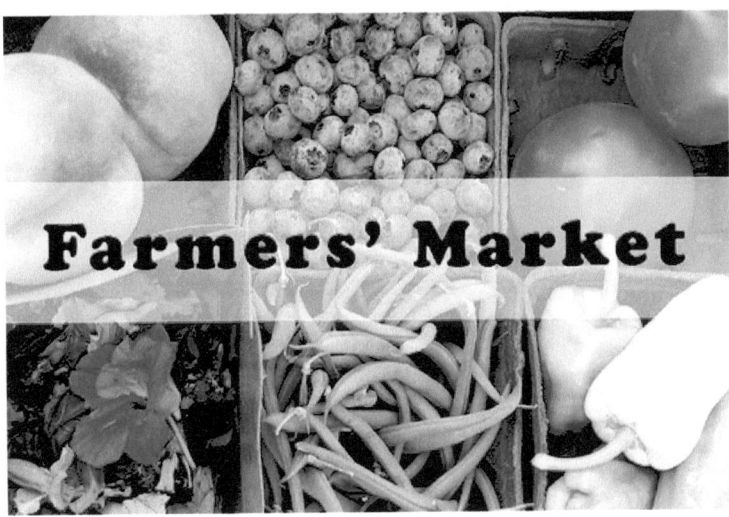

Still just want a quick fix and an unaltered lifestyle? Read on you will get what we promised.

So remember say "No, thank you"

to second servings, high sugared foods snacking, microwave, gluttony, processed food, fast food and fast eating, the 'feedbag', ...

So remember you can "add years to your life"

by eating 'slowly' raw and steamed

by going 'fermented' and 'nuts'

by enjoying it with 'moderation' & 'variation'

by sustaining your healthy behavior

by eating "**EnjoyVity**"

Always consult a dietician or doctor before making a major change in your diet and exercise routine.

6. Know how to drink

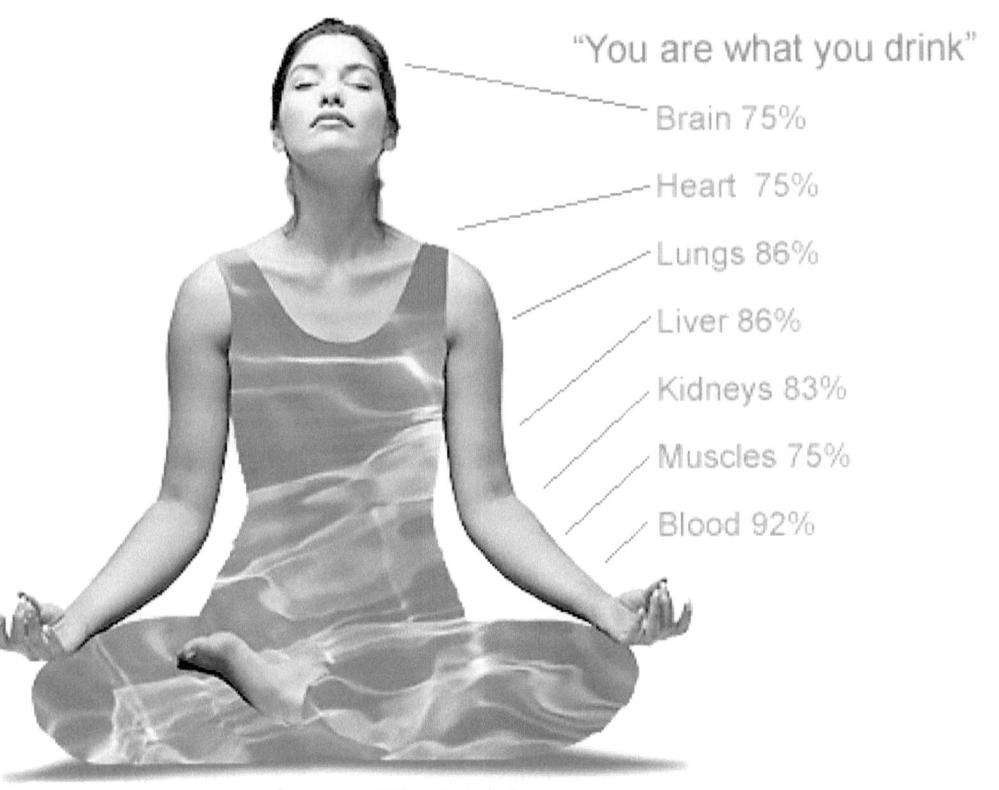

"You are what you drink"
Brain 75%
Heart 75%
Lungs 86%
Liver 86%
Kidneys 83%
Muscles 75%
Blood 92%

Your Body is 70% Water.

In order to maintain one's health and organ structure a human consumes approximately **25.000 liters of water** during the course of a lifetime. You have reasons to make the right choice.

...the way to avoid blood clotting is to drink more water, stop eating processed foods and work on relaxation techniques ...sounds like your grandmother's advice, right.

All life processes require the presence of water to function. The human metabolism functions optimally while taking sufficient pure and healthy water. If you have a balanced food intake with sufficient fresh fruit and vegetables you can consume less water.

If not 'pure' water, any drink should be considered as food, so use with moderation and enjoy, chew it, taste it, mix with your saliva to start the pre-digestion by help of enzymes already in your mouth. Do not just blindly swallow your drinks as it will be the start of over-consumption and insufficient assimilation.

Water why and how much: your body on average excretes 2.5 liter water a day through lungs (20%), skin (20%), feces (4%) and urine (56%). A shortness of 1 to 2% of body-water will give us pain and feel thirsty. You should thus add a similar (90%, remainder is own made metabolic water) amount daily through food and mainly drinking. Rule of thumb, one liter /30 kilo (1 quart/66 pounds) of body weight is needed on daily base. A professional endurance sportsman just as a deep underground mine worker will need liters (quarts) per working-hour not per day. Keep in mind the more your urine is colored the more your body lacks water. Your thirsty feeling comes always way too late as many universal studies indicated. Drink thus upfront to avoid cell damage or any disorder in one or more of the below related functions.

Remember that your 'water needs' equal your 'water desire' + 1/3.

If you have a hunger feeling there is great chance you are dehydrated. Thirst is often mistaken for hunger because the thirst mechanism is so weak. So grab a glass of good water before feeling hungry and certainly before feeling thirsty.

Functions of water in your body:

- Free our cells through lymph and blood from all breakdown and ballast products and as such protect you against degenerative sicknesses
- Let the kidneys fulfill their task optimally so that kidney- and bladder stones and insufficiencies are omitted
- Clean continuously the digestive system in order not to make gall stones and avoid constipation
- Help to control the body temperature
- The intercellular water acts as a buffer against seasonal diseases
- Avoid bone calcification, prevent joint blocking, stiffness and arthritis
- Help prevent eye cataract, brain calcification and tooth decay
- Prevent excess fluid retention and as such oedema formation, cellulites and obese
- Keep you lifelong flexible, healthy, fit and happy

> "Water is invaluable by what it carries and not by what it brings"
> ~Prof. Huchard

Which water to drink? Go for 'pure', meaning bacteria, cyst and virus free, and with as less minerals as possible. The mineral content can be found as TDS in milligram/liter. Prefer bottled water with <u>less</u> than **100 mg/l** total dissolved solids (mineral salts). Well and tap waters need further treatment before consumption due to potential presence of unknown or harmful substances. Additives in tap water like chlorine, a super-oxidant, have their meaning during transport but not in your body. Fluor, another super-oxidant, should not be dosed in your tap water! Keep your IQ up, get informed and take action: 'fluoridealert.org' !
So purify your drinking water at home with a professional kitchen filter like a under the sink reverse osmosis system (RO(*)), which will bring down the TDS to healthy levels and block all known and unknown taste, smells and substances from your drinking water. You assimilate organically bound minerals through your healthy food. Your drinking water should be '*empty*' of minerals so it can clean your metabolism. To your health!
(*) Get informed first and read the detailed information on BEV-certified reverse osmosis systems at 'purewatersystems.com' .

"BEV-standards water is the single most important nutrient for your body. Good water is also the most important component of any detox program. Put good things into your body = nutrition, get bad things out = detoxification. BEV-water is the foundation of both sides of this equation. Drinking BEV water has been one of the most valuable assets to my clients over the years, I would be hard pressed to find a modality that could provide greater benefit." ~ Dr. Robert B. Stephan BS, DDS, FAPD.

Bio-energize your purified water: make for instance a **'nettle'** tea (10' at 90C) based on purified or low mineral bottled water or add some drops of 'nettle' tincture. The nettle leaves hold high levels of minerals, especially, calcium, magnesium, iron, potassium, phosphorous, manganese, **silica**, iodine, silicon, sodium, and sulfur. They also provide chlorophyll and tannin, and they're a good source of vitamin C, beta-carotene, and B complex vitamins. Nettles also have high levels of easily absorbable amino acids. They hold ten percent protein, more than any other vegetable. Many of the benefits from the plant will be transferred to your nourishing herbal tea, such as its blood cleaning and re-mineralizing effects, but now with bio-absorbable organically bound minerals. Whenever you feel run down, tired, or even irritable, make some. You can also make a 'maseration' while keeping the leaves overnight in cold water. In spring your can also make nettle soup with your purified water as base. Easier is to add the "Ferments of Life" which will saturate your drinking water with **free electrons**. If added to your 'reverse osmosis' purified tapwater it will not only re-vitalize it, but lead its parameters towards the slightly acidic and anti-oxidizing 'terrain'(environment) of life enhancement, a true biocompatible drinking water. Find details at 'enjoyvity.com/the-7-pillars-of-the-lesik-ferments-of-life' or ask at 'sales@fermentsoflife.com'.

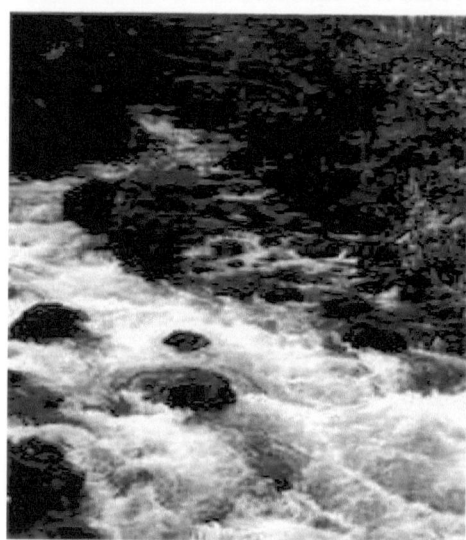
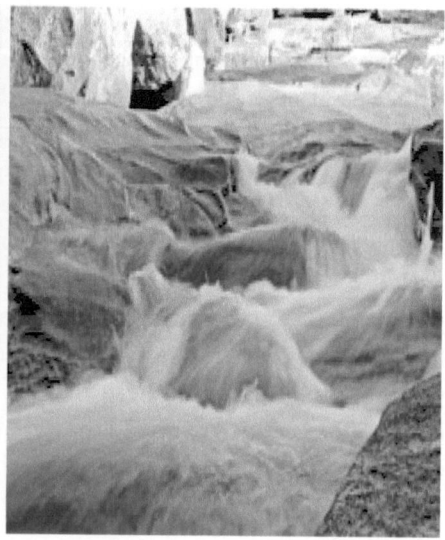

Listen to the force of water 'fengshui-consultants.co.uk'

Alkalized-Ionized water, yes or no: invented in the 50-ies by Russian scientists and globalized through Japan(*), Korea and the USA, made by electrolyses from tap water, its electrochemical parameters pH 9.5 and ORP -350 make it an exception of a kind (**). Flushes redundant acids out of the bodies 'mesenchym', but that is an illness situation, which can and should be measured and confirmed at first by an experienced physician (read page 76). Indeed are many other modern degenerative diseases defined by an acid extracellular 'terrain' in which case this unbalanced 'microwater' taken in quantities on daily base would cause at the end a worsening of the 'terrain'. Use with caution, consider it as a food supplement or an ailment to redirect the 'terrain' of certain patients. As confirmed by: "This artificial anti-oxidizing water has *not one* characteristic of a natural drinking water. If you are searching for anti-oxidizing properties you can as well drink a carrot juice or a good glass of red bio-wine." From 'Purify your table water/Purifiez votre eau de table" R.Haas, Edit. Trajectoire,2009

Also the idea that one must consume 'alkaline' water and minerals to neutralize the effects of acidic foods is scientifically untrue. We get rid of excess acid from metabolism by exhaling carbon dioxide (lungs) and by excreting urea acid (kidneys). Further are there many other reasons and solutions to become or stay balanced. If you do drink alkaline water, its alkalinity is quickly removed by the highly acidic gastric fluid in the stomach.

(*)Dr. Yoshiaki Matsuo PhD., the inventor of the *Japanese* Ionized Water unit stated: 'Ionized Water with its reduction potential of -250 to -300 mV is beyond comparison due to its ability to scavenge active oxygen radicals'. Also Sanetaka Shirahata's, Professor Cellular Regulation Technology, at the Kyushu University, Japan, research focused on the role of "active hydrogen," atomic hydrogen found in electrolyzed reduced water, in eliminating active oxygen and confirmed that this helps protect DNA from damage caused by oxidation.

(**) In nature it is almost impossible to find such outspoken and alkali and reduced water at a source or spring. The parameters promote the growth of bacteria as in waste water. Follow nature where all body-alkalizing fruits and vegetables have an acid pH to start with. The well intended advisors of **'alkaline water'** should understand that not one healthy food they support has these extreme parameters (pH+9, ORP-350 which equals an $rH_2>10$)!

Anyhow Dr. Hidemitsu Hayashi, heart specialist and director of the Water Institute of Japan in Tokyo, early defender of the 'ionized/alkaline water' theory and inventor of the recently marketed 'Hydrogen rich water stick', now remarks that: "alkaline, ionized water qualities in order of importance are: hydrogen, ORP, then alkalinity" and "If the body had all of the available hydrogen it needed, ORP and alkalinity would not matter- you would not need to consider it."

The health conscious should use daily a mineral-poor, slightly acidic and reduced drinking water as found in nature and stressed on earlier pages. Use the here discussed strongly alkaline and reducing waters only temporarily and under supervision! Moderation will be key, also here as we are looking to stay in balance not to get into new maybe different troubles.

Functional water can also be made with help of the organic Lesik®-ferments (*). The major and so important difference being that it will have next to its very strong reducing capabilities a natural slightly acidic pH and high resistivity.

(*) 'Free electrons' are here also the live saving and enhancing messengers (read chapter 8).

While referring to glacier water as in the 'Hunza' or any high mountain area one should understand that the parameters like the pH and rH2 are different at those very low temperatures and genuine locations then in your kitchen. The 'Hunza' did not drink just their water they were fully in balance with their environment; read further on it in chapter 11.

Yes, **you are what you drink**, also. About 21 percent of calories consumed by Americans over the age of 2 come from beverages, predominantly soft drinks and fruit drinks with added sugars. Add the current passion for smoothies and sweetened coffee drinks (there are 240 calories in a 16-ounce Starbucks Caffe Mocha without the whipped cream), and you can see why people are drinking themselves into XXXL sizes. In general beverages have "weak satiety properties" — they do little or nothing to curb your appetite — and people do not compensate for the calories they drink by eating less.

On top off, Barry Popkin, who directs an obesity program at the University of North Carolina, believes that: **"because we evolved drinking only water and getting all of our calories from food, liquid foods don't 'register' on our brain's appetite center the way solid foods do"**.

For example, a study by Harvard researchers found that **each** additional 12-ounce soft drink consumed per day increases the risk of a child becoming obese by 60 percent. For adults, the association is similar.
Here's a quick glance at the average daily consumption (per person) of liquid calories in a U.S. diet:

- Soda and sugary drinks: 203 calories
- Alcohol: 99 calories
- Milk: 84 calories
- 100% fruit-juice: 32 calories
- Coffee/tea: 11 calories

Milk, coffee, tea, herbal drinks, cacao, juices and alcohol

Milk: cow-milk is intended for new born veal's and even then for a short period in their life so limit the use of your traditional dairy products (whatever the marketing around them might tell you).
Also it is only since 120 years that we are sterilizing and pasteurizing. All our ancestors and the centenarian communities only used raw milk or milk products and even many times products based on fermented raw milk and in very limited amounts compared to the actual over-dosage.
A HUGE difference!

Soya-milk (actually soya-nut-juice): NO, non-fermented soy products can cause a variety of health problems if consumed in large quantities on a regular basis. Go for fermented soy products!
Further consider that since 1994, a growing number of foods were developed using

genetic modification (GMO). With these products has come controversy. Health concerns include: allergy, gene transfer (antibiotic-resistant genes from GMO to bacteria), and outcrossing (the movement of genes from GMO plants into conventional crops).**GMO soy** - About 90% of the American soybean crop planted today carries a gene that makes it resistant to an herbicide (Roundup, or glyphosate) used to control weeds and its use is rapidly growing throughout the world. GM-soy is estimated to be present in up to 70% of all food products found in US supermarkets, including cereals, breads, soymilk, pasta and most meat (as animals are fed GM-soy feed).

Kefir: fermented milk a great alternative, known and proven since millenaries for his freshness and health benefits like the suppressing of an increase in blood pressure and reducing of serum cholesterol levels.

Coffee: a modern approach, use it moderately. Several studies have linked regular coffee consumption to a reduced risk of developing Type 2 diabetes, colorectal cancer and Parkinson's disease. A study of more than 600 men suggested that drinking three cups of coffee a day protects against age-related memory and thinking deficits. Caffeine is a diuretic, it encourages the kidneys to produce urine so effectively that it may contribute to mild dehydration.

Tea: black or green since 10.000 years but remember always without milk as the protective effect that tea has on the cardiovascular system is totally wiped out by adding milk. White, green, oolong, and black teas all come from the leaves of the Camellia sinensis plant. They all stand for sharpening our concentration, help relieve diarrhea and lowers cholesterol levels.

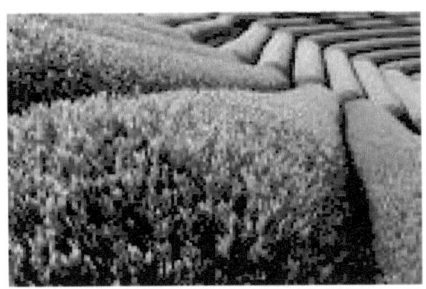
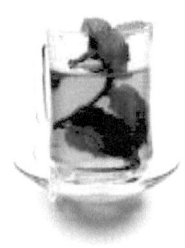

Black: made from fully fermented mature leaves. The compounds contained in black tea - theaflavins and thearubigens - do more than contribute to its dark color and distinctive flavor. They also provide health benefits originally attributed solely to green tea. Researchers concluded that the flavonoids in black tea helped reduce the production of LDL - the "bad" cholesterol that can lead to stroke and heart attacks. Furthermore, men who drank over four cups of black tea per day had a significantly lower risk of stroke than men who drank only two to three cups per day. 'Earl grey' tea for instance is made by combining quality black teas with the essential oil of the bergamot fruit, an orange-like fruit grown in the Mediterranean.

Green: What sets green tea apart is the way it is processed, namely made from steamed and dried mature leaves. The secret of green tea lies in the fact it is rich in bitter catechin polyphenols, the EGCG's, powerful antioxidants. The steaming of the leave prevents the EGCG compound from being oxidized. Green tea contains moderate amounts of caffeine, thus less than coffee. While searching for the health benefits drink 4 to 6 cups or more a day. Some of the features of EGCG's are the slowing of the aging process, lowering blood sugar, controlling high blood pressure, preventing the increase of cholesterol, practicing good oral hygiene, reducing the risk of cancer and preventing food poisoning. Cheers.

White: It are fresh buds or young leaves who are just lightly steamed and dried. Tea once reserved for the Emperor of China or visiting heads of state. These teas preserve much of the essence of the leaf, yielding a light sweet cup rich in healthy properties. Its caffeine content is only 10 to 15 mg, but its polyphenol content the highest.

Oolong: also called 'wulong' is made of partially fermented mature leaves and thus sits between green and black tea. Oolong tea burns 1.57 times more calories than green tea found Japanese researchers at the Tokushima University. Further is said that two cups of Oolong tea every day not only helps shed stubborn pounds by boosting your metabolism but also blocks the fattening effects of carbohydrates; promotes strong, healthy teeth; improves cognitive functioning and mental well-being; clarifies your skin, giving it a healthy, radiant glow and strengthens your immune system. Oolong has half the caffeine of green tea.

Experiments have shown that green tea after a first 5 minute brew contains 32 mg caffeine. But if the same leaves are then used for a second and then a third five minute brew, the caffeine drops to 12 mg and then 4 mg. Coffee brewed from grounds contains 40 mg/100ml , Expresso coffee 212 mg/100ml and Instant coffee 26 mg/100ml.

Coffee or tea as antidote for overdose of iron: Just like lead, mercury, cadmium, nickel, aluminum and other heavy metals, stored iron produces destructive free radicals. Recently, as said earlier, the iron content of food has been identified as the major life-shortening factor, rather than the calories. [Choi and Yu, Age vol. 17, page 93, 1994.] Iron causes cell aging, heart disease and cancer.

Thus our nutritional recommendations for iron have to be revised sharply downward. You should look for "ferrous" or "ferric" or "iron" on the label, and avoid foods with any added iron. Coffee, when taken with food, strongly inhibits the absorption of iron, so try to drink coffee with meat. Also tea contains tannin, which blocks the absorption of iron.
At best **avoid over consumption of red meat.**

> **Rooibos:** also called red tea although it is made from a total different herb with his origins in South Africa. Rooibos is a flavorful (sweet and nutty), caffeine-free alternative to 'real' tea. Rooibos or 'redbush' is a naturaly green leaf which turns red when fermented. Rooibos is known to treat allergies, to assist with nervous tension, with digestive problems and for its anti-oxidant content bringing cardiovascular and anti-aging benefits. Its polyphenol content maybe half of that of green tea but searchers found already up to 11 different kinds. The low-in-tannin content of this herbal remedy will prevent that it turns bitter even after standing.

Herbal infusions:

> **Minth:** make a hot beverage infusion with menthol from real fresh peppermint leaves for overall digestion improvement. It is a good mouth and breath freshener, and providing symptommatic relief for painful inflammatory states like arthritis, chronic tendinitis, and acute sprains and strains. Mint is also a good to help relaxation and can be used in nervous con ditions, for stress, anxiety and sleeplessness. Infusion is mostly made in combination with green tea.

> **Ginkgo Biloba:** with an aging population seeking solutions to troubling problems such as dementia ginkgo offers some benefit. The leaf extract is the most widely sold phytomedicine in Europe, where it is used to treat the symptoms of early-stage Alzheimer's disease, vascular dementia and age-related cognitive decline others. It also is one of the 10 best-selling herbal medications in the United States. Recently however researchers at the Virginia University found that it is ineffective Against Dementia, (10/2008).

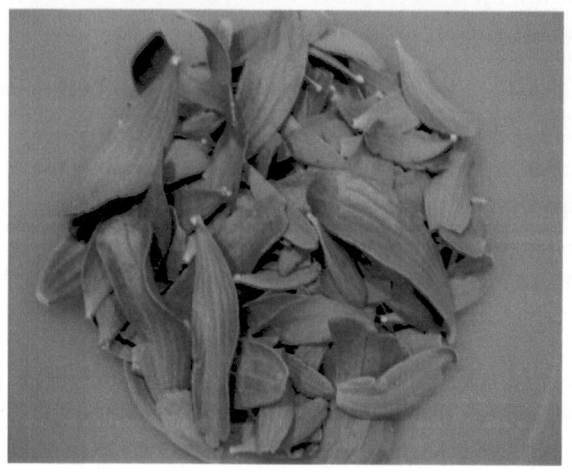

Mistletoe: the twigs and leaves are a heart tonic, reduce blood pressure, slow heart rate, strengthen capillary walls, against ear buzz, stimulate the immune system and inhibit tumors.

Make a cold 'maseration' (+8 hrs) of the leaves and drink 2 cups (lukewarm if preferred) a day for +2 weeks.

Hibiscus: known for its cholesterol and blood pressure reducing effects. Drink it as such or combined with wild rose or your own favorite herb.

Green mate: a traditional beverage in South America, consisting of unfermented leaves of Ilex paraguariensis. Mate holds caffeine and promotes energy, and recently demonstrated to improve fatty acid oxidation.

Want to know **more about herbs** and things with Dr. Michael James 'the Reality of Herbal therapy: 'drugfreehelp.com'.

Fruit-and vegetable juices: a must, try pomegranate-, blackberry-, grape-....- or mulberry juices. The darker the better. They are loaded with antioxydants (see also "Never say no to *NO*" from Nobel prizewinner Dr. Lou Ignarro). They are also a *sweet* alternative, although not nearly as good as, whole fruits, which are better at satisfying hunger. In need for exclusive and healthy juices search also: florahealth.com and find the benefits of haw-thorn, nettle, St John's wort, valerian, dandelion, artichoke and even black radish.

Soft drinks: No, only exceptional! Mind their fructose content.

Cacao: Dr. N. Hollenberg of Harvard Medical School found that Kuna Indians, who live on the San Blas Island Chain in Panama and drink high quantities of cocoa drinks, have a much lower risk of stroke, heart failure, cancer and diabetes compared to the Indians living on the mainland. They can drink up to 40 cups of cocoa a week. The compound correlated to the findings is epicatechin and belongs to the group of the flavonols. High quantities of epicatechin can be found thus in cocoa, but also in blueberries, tea and grapes. Make your **cacao drink with water** not with milk as chocolate milk blunts the effects of the catechins (the powerful anti-oxidants that fight against cancer-causing cells and help prevent heart disease) in the chocolate, similar as when adding milk to your tea.

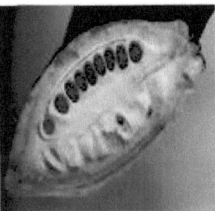 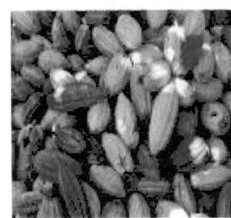 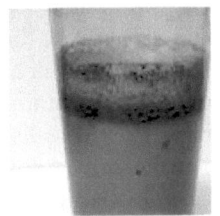 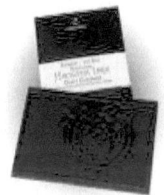

By deduction we can state that milk chocolate is also no comparison for + 70% true black chocolate when your body is searching for anti-oxidants, vitamins or endorphines. Researchers found that chocolate - specifically dark chocolate - contains 53.5 mg of catechins per 100 grams. By contrast, 100 ml of black tea contains a mere 13.9 mg of catechins.

Alcohol how and when: Alcohol, fermented and distilled drinks are of all civilizations. Avoid abuse; don't drink on your own. Keep it a social event and know your own limits, don't try to match up with others.

Don't mix with oxygen! Vodka+olive oil (15%) to protect stomach.

Mind the '**BAC**' (blood alcohol content) calculator :
Alcohol leaves the body of virtually everyone at a constant rate of about .015 percent of blood alcohol content (BAC) per hour. Thus, a person with a BAC of .015 would be completely sober in an hour while a person with a BAC of ten times that (.15) would require 10 hours to become completely sober. This is true regardless of sex, age, weight, and similar factors.

Drink alcohol regularly but with 'moderation'. Moderate consumption of alcohol appears to be beneficial to reducing or preventing many diseases and health problems. Consuming alcohol in moderation reduces the risk of heart disease dramatically. It also significantly reduces the risk of stroke and other major causes of death. And evidence of the overall health benefits of moderate drinking continues to grow.

The best choice among the alcoholic drinks is then **red wine** due to, but not only, its resveratrol content. This brings us to the "**French Paradox**".

For years, researchers were puzzled by the fact that, despite consuming a diet rich in fat, the French have a lower incidence of heart disease than Americans. The answer was found to lie in red wine, which contains resveratrol, a polyphenol that limits the negative effects of smoking and a fatty diet.

The **resveratrol** antioxidant may decrease the development of some cancers and affects the immune system and inflammation in the body; both components are thought to be important in the development of plaque buildup in blood vessels, which often leads to heart disease.
Red wine also contains tannins, which may raise HDL (good) cholesterol levels and inhibit platelet cells in the blood from clumping together. Also in this type of wine can be found saponins, antioxidants believed to promote heart health by binding to cholesterol in the blood and preventing its absorption and may play a role in decreasing inflammation.

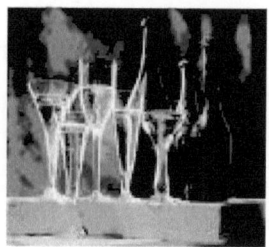 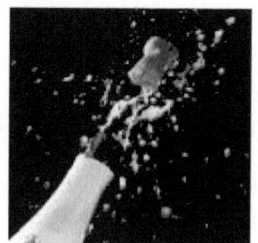 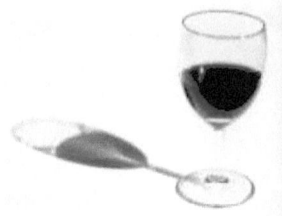

Show them you are "Enjoyvity": drink or better smell your wine from a brandy glass.

Search for best organic or **Bio**-wines which even smell much better than they taste. This will make it   easier for you to stay with that first glass.

If you never drank wine, then don't start. Better drink dark, purple **grape juice** it will hold the same polyphenols as in red wine.

Champagne: CHEERS, this exclusive beverage can help protect the brain against neurological injuries   that are obtained during a stroke. It also protects the brain from the degenerative effects of Alzheimer's and Parkinson's disease. The reason champagne is a health benefit is because of the high level of polyphenols that are found in it. These are antioxidants that assist in avoiding cell death when   there is a presence of oxidative stress. For a detailed story you can read 'the healing power of champagne' by dr.Kay & dr.Drouard, Savoir-Boire ltd 2006.

Also did we learn from the **Bioelectronic Vincent** (*) 'terrain' measurements that champagne has pronounced **'acid and reducing'** properties (see Bio-Electronic Health Diagram).
It was L.C. Vincent who demonstrated that our modern civilization induces an 'alkalization' of blood, and that it is essential to consume assimilable acids(read also chapt.5 under acid/alkaline foods). We find these also in wines, certainly in Champagne and good wines made following the 'method champenoise'!

As professor Louis-Claude Vincent said:
" Measure *the terrain* of an illness and deprive it of its breeding ground and the illness will heal by itself!"

(*) *'bevincent.com' Bioelectronics according to Vincent (BEV) is also defined as the science of biological fundamentals; it measures the electromagnetic currents that characterize life and standardizes them with three physical parameters: pH, rH2, r. Find examples of a BEV diagram page 95 and of an evaluation report under chapt.25.*

It was **Claude Bernard** who defined, 150 years ago, the term 'terrain' making its statement:
"**The terrain is everything; the germ is nothing**",
and then drank down a glass of water filled with cholera.
Louis Pasteur who went against it admitted on his deathbed to his friend Dr. Renon, that Bernard was right, but forbid his family to spread this knowledge. Pasteur with his **impostures** abused his colleagues and was followed by 20th century medicine (vaccinations) and industry (pasteurization) which ruined world health. Upon the death of Pasteur's grandson in 1975, 10,000 pages of laboratory notes became public. Then only it became clear that an entire century of medical history would have been different had the facts been presented as we now know them to have been.
It was definitely also about 'terrain', acid pH and cellular oxygen content, when Dr. Otto Warburg, in his 1966 lecture at the reception of his second Nobel Prize stated clearly: "**...nobody today can say that one does not know what cancer and its prime cause is. On the contrary, there is no disease whose prime cause is better known, so that today ignorance is no longer an excuse that one cannot do more about prevention.**"

"They" continue the **mandatory vaccination**, without questioning, but now is the "**ZeitGeist**' such that you GET the right information where it is available!
Like at here: '**sayingnotovaccines.com**'. "You expect that your doctor/pediatrician would at least explore the possibility that vaccine(s) played a role when your children regress after vaccination into poor health, autism, learning disabilities, ADD/ADHD, epilepsy, asthma, diabetes, arthritus, intestinal bowel disorders and many other kinds of brain and immune system dysfunction". Thank You Dr. Sherry Tenpenny your courage is worth quintillion's of pennies.

Great time thus for changing your 'environment'!

Definition of 'Terrain': all cells live in essentially the same environment, the extracellular fluid, for which reason the extracellular fluid is called the internal environment of the body, the 'milieu intérieur', a term introduced by French physiologist Claude Bernard.

The shift of the pathological terrain into a physiological terrain (substrate or environment) can be completed with the help of homeopathy, phytotherapy, and also allopathy or with the right choice of foods and drinks if the basics are clearly understood. For details: 'phmiracleliving.com', doctors only: 'oirf.com', or at our website 'enjoyvity.com/experts'.

Of course, not everyone should drink alcohol, including pregnant women, those who have ever experienced difficulty controlling their drinking, or anyone whose physician recommends abstinence.

Medical researchers generally describe 'moderation' as one to three drinks per day. Where, a typical woman should drink 25 to 30% less than an average man.

A drink is a 12 ounce/33 cc can or bottle of beer, a 5 ounce/140 gram glass of wine, or 1.5 ounces/40 gram of liquor (either straight or in a mixed drink). Each contains the same amount of alcohol -- six-tenths of an ounce/ 17gram and they are all the same to a breath-analyzer. Find a great visualization at 'standarddrinks.com'

What is then **moderate drinking**? The US government currently defines moderation for a woman as consuming no more than one drink per day and for men it is drinking no more than two drinks per day.

Many other countries define moderation at much higher levels of consumption. For example, in the Netherlands moderation is about three drinks per day for both men and women and in France it's about two and one-half drinks per day for women and over four drinks per day for men. Until recently, the US National Institute on Alcohol Abuse and Alcoholism defined moderation for men as consuming up to four drinks in a day.

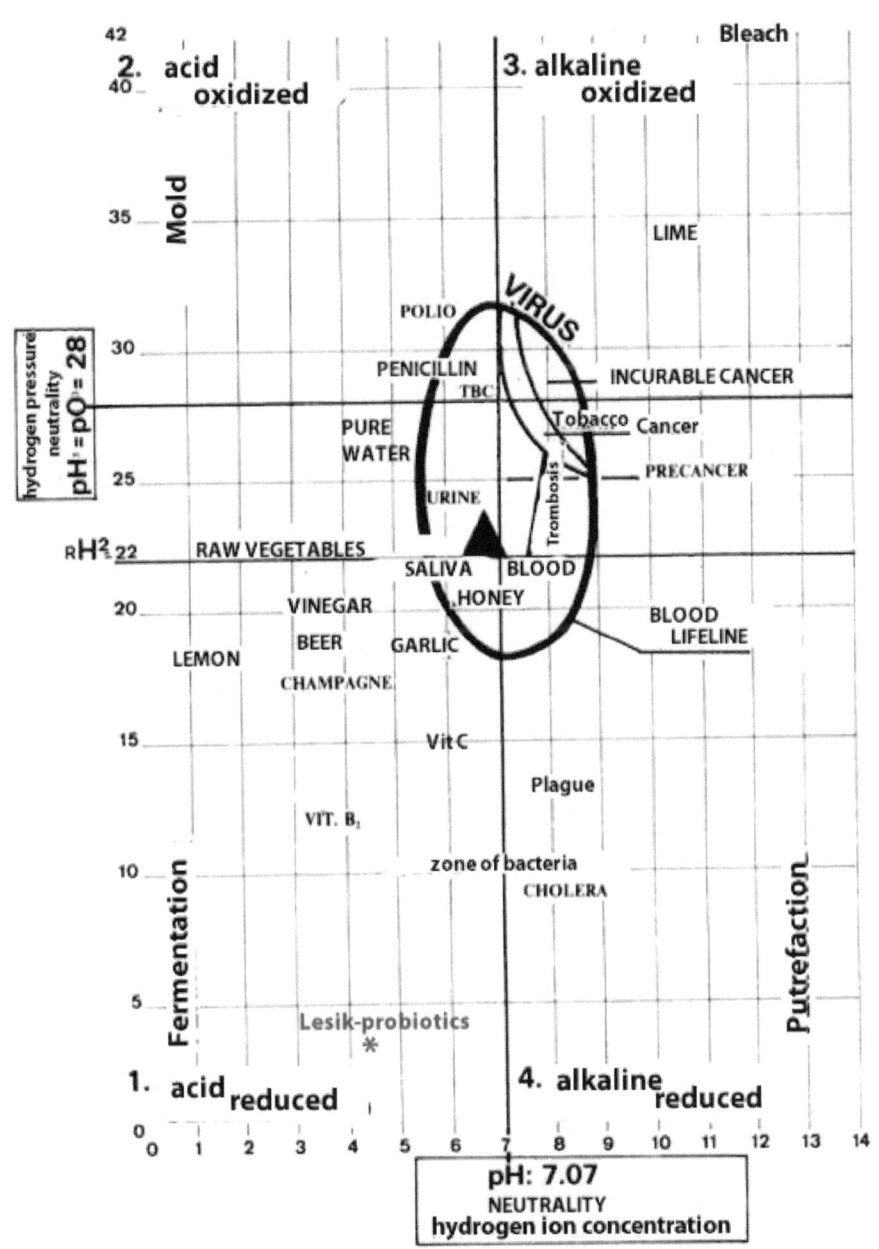

People need to **be aware** of some important medical facts about drinking:

- The risk of dying in any given year is 25 percent lower for those who consume moderate amounts of alcohol.
- Moderate drinking reduces the risk of stroke by about one-half.
- Moderate drinkers have a 54% lower chance of developing dementia than abstainers.
- Moderate drinkers are over 30-40 percent less likely to develop diabetes.

"The benefits of drinking in moderation begin early in life and they apply to beer, wine, and liquor or distilled spirits (gin, vodka, whiskey, tequila, rum, bourbon, etc.)" says David Hanson Professor Emeritus of Sociology at the State University of New York in Potsdam, New York. He has researched the subject of alcohol and drinking for over 30 years and has written widely on the subject (*while sponsored by the Alcohol mfg-association*).

In general, consumption of about 80 grams of 'absolute' alcohol daily for a significant length of time is required for men to develop ALD (alcohol and liver disease). 80 grams of alcohol is roughly equivalent to a six-pack of beer or a liter of wine. (To convert grams to ounces multiply by 20 and divide by 567.) Women are much more susceptible to the toxicity of alcohol than are men. It has been estimated that it takes as little as 20 grams of daily alcohol ingestion over an extended period of time for women to develop ALD. (see 'liverdisease.com').

Are you **addicted** to alcohol? Ask yourself the following 4 questions, known as the CAGE questions:

1. Have you tried to CUT down in your drinking?
2. Are you ANNOYED with criticisms about drinking?
3. Do you sometimes feel GUILTY about drinking?
4. Do you sometimes drink alcohol in the morning or as an "EYE-OPENER"?

If you answer "yes" to at least 2 of these questions, there is a 75% chance that you are addicted to alcohol. On the other hand, if you answer yes to just one question or to none of them, there is a 96% chance that you are not. Having a problem with alcohol will shorten your health span and will certainly decrease your quality of life. Seeking assistance and treatment is critical.

So remember say "No, thank you"
        to alcohol over-consumption

            to 'red' meat without coffee or tea

So remember you can add years to your life

by drinking +8 glasses of 'good' water/day

by drinking fruit- & veggie juices

by drinking a glass of red wine or champagne

by drinking white tea or cacao with water

7. Know how to look

People seldom notice old clothes if you wear a big smile. ~Lee Mildon

Do you have your own 'look'? If not define yours.

What is a 'look' about? Image? To look good!
Everyone knows that looks DO make a difference.
Clothes that fit your figure, shoes with a fresh shine, wrinkle-free knit shirt and pressed dress trousers, lipstick maybe, some perfume, hairstyle, ..., even a clean inside of your car. Get attention with a hat. Own a great pair of sunglasses. Eat balanced, drink enough pure water, breath consciously and exercise all this will make that your skin glows, you stretch your back and that your eyes sparkle.
Do you feel already more confident? It is all in the details. It starts from the inside.

What you think you look like? What is your self image?
Image is about how you 'see' yourself and how 'you' believe others see you.
But how do you 'feel' about yourself? Do you lack **self esteem**?
Self esteem is how much value you place on yourself and this includes your self-image, your personality, your job, relationships and many other factors. A high level of self esteem brings with it high self confidence.
No one's closer to you than you! Love yourself, from the inside out.
Avoid negative minded people or at least don't get absorbed by them.
Stand tall, go prepared, smile and believe in yourself.
Think positive and become a winner.

Help others to learn and grow, and support them in achieving their greater self-awareness. *Want to know more about building your self esteem, try: 'more-selfesteem.com'* .

It is about getting the other party to look, listen to you. Your hair, your clothing and your accessories should all be in tune to the tastes of the other party, be it your partner, colleague, boss or friend.
Meet your personality. Metamorphose, dear to change your wardrobe or combine in a different way.
Many of us are walking around with a less-than-flattering silhouette caused by an ill-fitting piece of clothing or even undergarment. Your clothes should flatter your body. Use natural fabrics that feel comfortable and great against your skin: silky satin, cotton, soft suede, wool or Cashmere. Avoid synthetics. People are increasingly wearing energetically „discharged„ clothing, thereby excluding a further opportunity for well-being. Get ideas but don't copy and don't follow just the ever-changing mode. Don't let then classify you as having only one style.
Style is about looking great no matter what you wear. If you feel not comfortable

in an outfit, don't buy. Only in comfortable clothes and shoes you can feel happy. Which makes you smile and people will like you.

You never get a second chance to make a first impression. Note that an important impression while meeting for first time is taken from the 20 cm of your face and your first 20 words spoken during the first 20 seconds.

20C20W20S and you are pre-bagged not only when in sales!

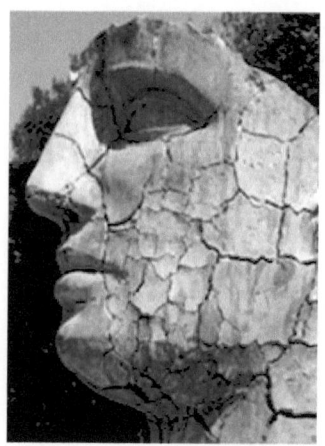

The first 20 cm: Some dermatologists now believe that almost three-fourths of all skin damage caused by the sun is caused prior to the time we turn 18. Full-body exercises will help improve blood and oxygen flow throughout the body, which will keep facial skin looking younger and healthier. Deep breathing will also help oxygenation your skin. Poor nutrition and especially excessive refined sugar will increase cellular aging and thus wrinkle formation. With aging our skin loses its flexibility. First anti-wrinkle advice: avoid sun damage while applying sunscreen and wear a hat against sun rays.

AGEs (advanced glycation end products) start damaging the proteins in the body, including the fibers known as collagen and elastin which are critical to healthy and young looking skin. Cut back drastically on **refined sugar**'s and reduce the development of 'AGEs' while adding plenty of foods that are low on the glycemic index (*). These foods would include whole grains, most fruits, vegetables, and many types of nuts.   Indeed
another piece of your same puzzle. The picture gets clearer and less complicated. Keep on smiling. They can even hear you smiling at the phone.

(*) For the **GI**, a ranking of carbohydrates on a scale from 0 to 100 according to the extent to which they raise blood sugar levels after eating, search: <u>glycemicindex.com</u> . Do it before getting filed by 3rd parties under 'diabetes'.

Anti wrinkle exercises for your face: If you want to give to your face the look that Yoga and Pilates can give to the body... - that young, elegant, balanced, firm look you should try facial exercises as the ones from Carolyn's Facial Fitness, CFF®, find 'carolynsfacialfitness.com' or look at her free DVD 'carolynsfacialfitness.com/dvd-clip' or give your neck a straight, gulping try here:

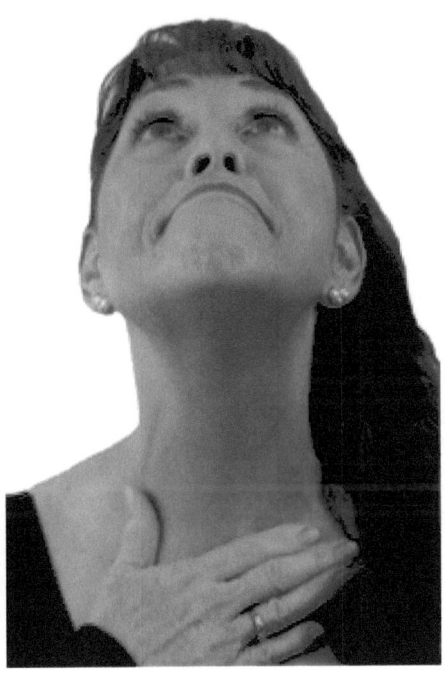

Gulping Fish: place your open hand at the base of your throat, stretched across your collarbone. Holding your hand down, extend your neck up, leading with your chin and stretch with your bottom jaw, only, towards the ceiling. Do NOT swallow, but rather reach with your bottom lip towards the ceiling "looking" like a gulping fish. Make 10 "gulps". Do 5 sets, changing hands for each round.

Wake up with a **big smile** on your face it will also increase your self esteem. Make thus smiling your preferred exercise. Mouth corners to your ears and eyebrows up, feel the difference. Now is the time to have a positive look at the world and live your dreams.

Smiling will gain you ten more years of life. ~Chinese proverb

Beauty from the inside out with Aloe! Of course you want to keep your innate, natural beauty for as long as you possibly can. Day lotions and night creams tick the sensory delight boxes of touch and smell, but for how long do they actually provide your skin with nutrients and antioxidants? A big leap up from lotions and creams are freshly prepared facial masks that contain Aloe. A quantum leap further still is **your bloodstream**, as the 24/7/365 source of nutrients and antioxidants, providing of course that you put these into your mouth and that they are absorbed.

Anti-Aging - three effective wrinkle remedies:

1- **Optimum Nutrition** - we know that electron-donating nutrition is the very basis of anti-ageing. You may achieve that via *plenty of raw foods* with dark green, red and purple colors.

2- **Minimum Pollution** - This is as much a theoretical no-brainer as it is a common practical pitfall.

3- **Accelerated Repair** - Nothing works better than a high quality Aloe supplement. Learn more and get your free e-book on naturally improved digestion: 'aloeride.eu'

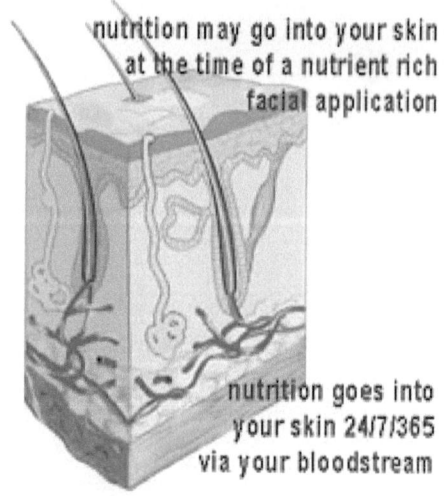

nutrition may go into your skin at the time of a nutrient rich facial application

nutrition goes into your skin 24/7/365 via your bloodstream

The first 20 seconds: People have prejudices remember and have a need to catalogue; we are animals who survived for millenaries by using our intuition our survival reactions. Your 'look' helps them to 'file' you in seconds. If you don't want to be 'deleted' in seconds, then you should get your 'look' right.

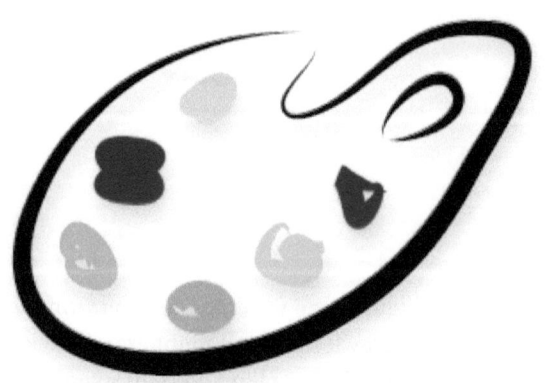

Color your day! Choose your pallet.

Be surrounded with Your color. Colors affect us psychologically. They can make us excited, happy, irritated, angry or sad. The right colors help you look younger, fresher and more vibrant. It is not because it is your favorite color that it is flattering to you. Put all type of colored pieces you find in your wardrobe close to your face and watch the result in the mirror, or go to a fabric shop and hold the different materials in front of you. The best colors leave you looking healthy, vibrant and refreshed. Take mental notes of the colors you are wearing when people compliment you.

The full spectrum of your 'look'

Red - means passion
Red is the warmest of all colors. It represents passion, energy, desire, excitement, love, strength, courage, leadership and power. Red reflects energy and can increase enthusiasm and interest. It enhances human metabolism, raises blood pressure and increases respiration rate.

Orange - means energy
Orange represents enthusiasm, fascination, success, attraction, encouragement, and determination. It is always associated with sunshine, joy and autumn. Curiosity is a driving characteristic of orange when it comes to explore new things. It is said that people who like orange are usually thoughtful and sincere.

Yellow - means joy
Yellow is always full of creative and intellectual energy. Yellow symbolizes wisdom, happiness, wealth, hope, cheerful, and intellect. It brings clarity for decision-making and awareness, sharper memory and concentration skills. Men usually perceive yellow as a very 'childish' color.

Green - means nature
It symbolize the master healer, well being, life, fertility, freshness, ambition, growth, stability and endurance. It is the most restful color for the human eye. Dark green is always associated with money, banking, and the financial world. Green is a safe, universal color.

Blue - means peace
Blue is the coolest color. It represents calm, truth, loyalty, wisdom, confidence, intelligence, faith, harmony, heaven, sincerity and trust. Blue is considered beneficial to the mind and body which slows down human metabolism and produces a calming effect. Blue also symbolizes conservatism, coldness and depression. Blue is highly accepted among males. Dark blue is associated with expertise and stability.

Black - means stability
Black is the most misunderstood color. Black is a mysterious color associated with fear and the unknown. It is also associated with power, elegance, formality, death and evil. Black is considered to be a very formal, elegant and prestigious color. It contrasts well with bright colors.

Purple - means power
It is associated with royalty. Purple symbolizes luxury, ambition, magic and mystery, inspirational and imagination. It is also a color of good judgment.

Being the combination of red and blue, the warmest and coolest colors, purple is most favored by children.

White - means purity
It means cleanliness, innocent, goddess and safety. It is considered to be the color of perfection.

Gray - means neutrality
Gray is the color of sorrow. It is the symbol for security, maturity, dependability and reliability.

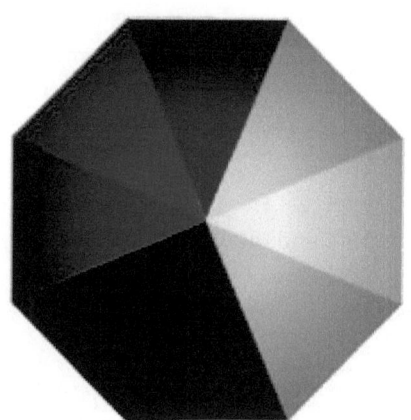

Knowing what range of colors suit you best and how to skillfully coordinate them will make you appear younger, healthier, more professional, people friendly and energized. Try complementary colors, which are opposite each other on the color wheel. **Choose now** the colors for Your personality & life goals. Search further: 'colourtherapyhealing.com'.

Build your image. Feel free to make mistakes. Or Re-look with a coach.

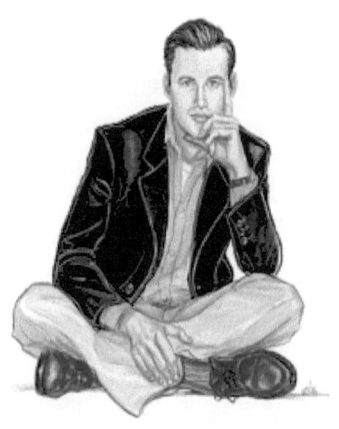
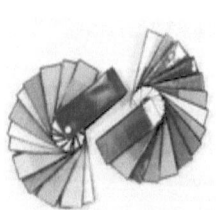
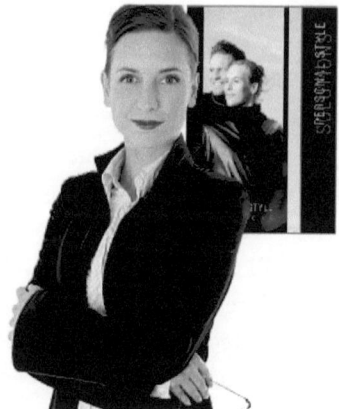

Need help in defining and creating your new look? Get free information and get it done online: 'taic.com.au'

Feng Shui and clothing: it affects not only the way you feel, but can influence your destiny. For more search:: 'fashionfengshui.com' and read 'Dressing the Whole Person, Nine Ways to Create Harmony & Balance in Your Wardrobe (& Prosperity in Your Life!)', the first book to link fashion and Feng Shui." By Evana Maggiore 'thefabricofourlives.com'

Slow down, take care of the new YOU. Get out of the grey as if you must, move into the sun because you want. Enjoy that new part of your puzzle of life.
Reach for **the full "EnjoyVity" spectrum.**

Need still an outside view, a helping hand, someone coaching you through your life goals, so you look better from the inside out.
Get your 24/7 personal coach. A great personal development coach is a sounding board, helps with motivation and goal setting and achievement, work life balance, quality of life, interpersonal skills, communication support, self image and self appreciation so that you get the maximum return on YOU. Make your choice, light your fire: 'coach-companion.com' or self improve with help of an expert 'selfgrowth.com/experts.html'.

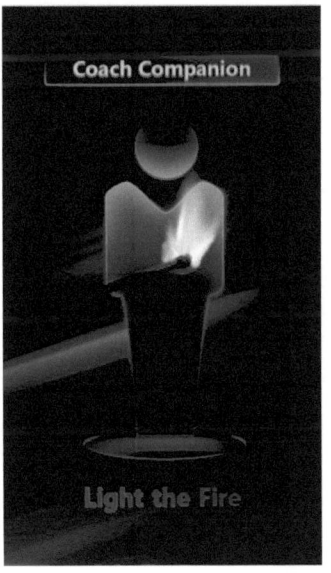

So remember say "No, thank you"
> to wrinkles

>> to uncomfortable clothes

So remember you can add years to your life
> by feeling confident

> by smiling

> by reaching for the

>> **full spectrum of your life**

8. Know how to clean-up

Take care of your body. It's the only place you have to live. ~Jim Rohn

Our body is made up of over 600 trillion (*) cells. Cells are constantly being born and dying and cells have different life spans ranging from hours to years. So you change your skin every month!

LIFESPAN OF SOME CELLS IN THE HUMAN BODY	
Granulocytes	10 hours to 3 days
Stomach lining cells	2 days
Sperm cells	2-3 days
Colon cells	3-4 days
Skin epidermal cells	2 - 4 weeks
Red blood cells	4 months
Endothelial cells	months – years
Pancreas cells	1 year or more
Bone Cells	25 - 30 years

But there is more in and around our body. Many trillions of tiny organisms, bacteria, viruses, and fungi live on our skin and in our mouths and guts. The latest estimation speaks of **60 trillion bacteria** in our gut only. The Harvard School of Dental Medicine, have found **6 billion** and 615 different species of 'salivary' bacteria in our mouth- and they're still counting. Remember--in a healthy mouth, most microbes help keep each other in balance. You better choose a mild natural toothpaste without aggressive chemicals and oxidants like Fluor to take care of your needed flora and the **digestive enzymes** in your saliva. As we age, our body loses its ability to produce its own enzymes. So we have to include them in our diet, by eating raw (cooking destroys them) organic (without preservatives) food. Good food sources for enzymes are most ripe fruits, vegetables, nuts and sea vegetables. More important details on your digestion from Stephney A. Langford: 'jigsawhealth.com/pdf'

(*) Get your trillion right

Français	British English	American English
milliard	milliard	billion
billion	billion	trillion
trillion	trillion	quintillion

Thus an American trillion equals 1000 billion or a million millions or 10 to the power of 12 (short scale), while on the European continent a trillion equals 10 to the power of 18 (long scale). The 600 trillion cells of our body could equal thus 6 x (10 to the power of 14) and in Europe we would better name it then 600 billion. There is still some dispute among scientist as many say that our body contains over 200 quintillion cells; this would mean that the 600 trillion figure we find all over in medical papers is referring to the European/long scale trillion and in the US we should speak about 200 or 600 (what's in a figure) quintillion.

Some more figures for the fun: until recently, astronomers estimated that the Big Bang occurred between 12 and 14 billion years ago. To put this in perspective, our Solar System is thought to be 4.5 billion years old and humans have existed as a species for a few million years. Astronomers also estimate that there are 70 sextillion stars in the 'visible' universe, or some 70 thousand million million million. That's a 7 followed by 22 zeros or (10 to the 22nd power, as used in the long scale system of numeration).

Our* 'Milky Way' galaxy is a gravitationally bound collection of roughly two hundred billion stars. Our Sun is one of these stars and is located roughly 24,000 light years (just under ten trillion kilometers/~6 trillion miles) from the center of our galaxy. Alpha Centauri and Proxima Centauri, the stars nearest our solar system, are about 4.3 light-years distant. The Milky Way measures 100.000 lightyears across. Try to visualize this! A 'light second', the distance travelled by light through a vacuum in a second, is 186,000 miles or 300,000 kilometers. So light needs just $1/20^{th}$ of a second to make it say from London to Los Angeles. You can watch many stars tonight by their ancient light which is travelling to us while the stars itself may no longer exist.

* A new infra red digital survey of the entire sky was made in 2003. Teams from the universities of Virginia and Massachusetts used a supercomputer to sort through half a billion stars to create a new star map showing our Solar System (dot on the left) to be at the exact nexus crossroads where two galaxies are actually joining. We are from another galaxy, the Sagittarius Dwarf galaxy, in the process of joining with the Milky Way. The Milky Way is actually not our parent galaxy!

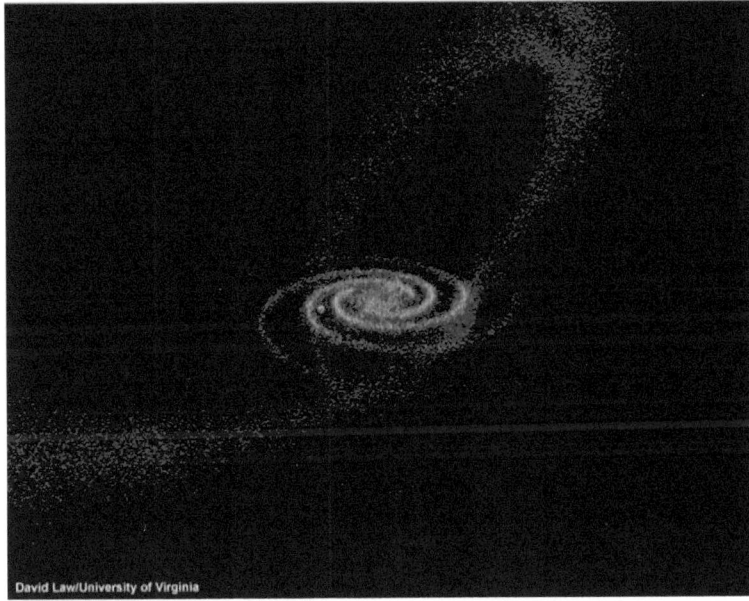

Maybe time for some to re-evaluate some of Velikovsky's theories.

The Hubble Space Telescope has found there may be 125 billion galaxies in the, or better 'our', universe, as there may be something like a '**megaverse**'.

The Carina nebula, about 7,500 light-years away, reveals glowing dust and brilliant star clusters

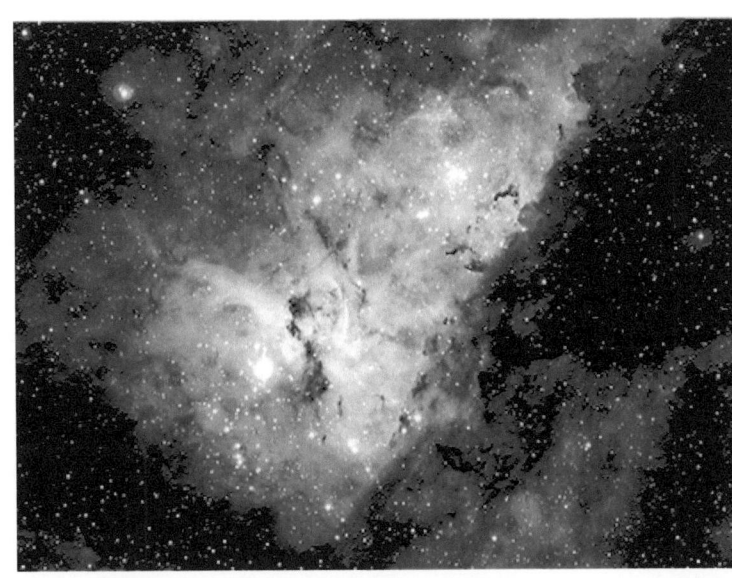

The world's population, estimated at 200 million in the year 1, is today (07-2010) about 6.9 billion and will reach 15 billion (or milliard in the long scale) by just 2040!

Best relatives, as with figures you can prove anything, right. Also most official figures given are average figures about average persons. We want you to avoid to be considered and "average". What does it tell you that within the same life expectancy figures sits that 95 year old true healthy person and another nonagenarian who is partly dement and deadly sick. Right we are in for **'quality of life'**.

'EnjoyVity' equals *'enjoying a vital lifestyle and good health into our very old age.'*

Let us step down from our throne and get some cleaning action to slow our aging in a youthful way!

A healthy body can cure a sick mind and a healthy mind can cure a sick body. Where to start?

So back to our body and its largest organ: **the skin**. Under normal circumstances, every minute of the day we lose about 30,000 to 40,000 dead skin cells off the surface of our skin - that's about 4 kilograms per year of dead skin cells (and that is again an average). In fact, much of the dust in a house is to a great extent comprised of our dead skin cells. Daily skin cleaning will keep the skin clean and the dead skin cell layer to a healthy minimum.

Use good brushes and combine dry brushing of your whole body before and wet brushing during your shower.

A room temperature of 20C/68F is for some people warm for others fresh. You can and best should bring down your skin comfort threshold. Combine cold shower with a hot finish style sauna, use a **Kuhne** ice packing, do your Kneipp coldwater stepping, walk naked in-home, lower your room temperature (in steps of 1c/1.8F towards 18C/64.4F) and avoid AirCo (all great for your budget, feeling and our environment). A lower skin and body temperature will increase your metabolism.

Daily showers, a bath maybe and Kneipp, Kuhne, herbal infusion's for sure

Kneipp: Sebastian Kneipp revolutionized naturopathic medicine in the 19 century. According to Kneipp, it is the combination of all four elements: water, plants, exercise and diet that keeps body, mind and soul in balance. Hot and cold rinses, knee and thigh rinses, cold rinses, cold footbaths (15-20 seconds) and water stepping. An example of a short morning 'Kuhr" in the shower (after a warm shower for instance): with cold water (max 18C) move your showerhead from right foot till top of outside right leg return from the inside of right leg, switch to left foot and up and down, same from right hand to right shoulder from outside return from right arm inside to hand and switch to left hand up and down, start from pubis in circles up body till neck and back down finish with head and face. Enjoy your day: 'kneipp.com' and 'kneippus.com'.

Take the test and check your Toxicity Level and learn about the *Grassroots Solutions for Modern Health Concerns* while participating in the Health Quiz: 'florahealth.com'.

The Kuhne Detox Bath's: working principle is to refresh (*) the core area of the body, around the groin and genitals with cold re-usable gel packages (the modern way) or cold water 'diversion frictions' (as initiated by Louis Kuhne over 100 years ago in Switzerland) during 10 minutes daily or longer, depending on your initial condition, and the results you seek to achieve. This process creates a vibration in the fascia, the interconnecting tissue covering all internal organs, which sets in motion a roll-back effect that transports digestion's leftover fats and deposited toxins back to the intestines, where they are later eliminated.

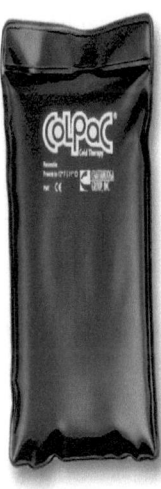

Results: Detox, stabilization of weight and later weight loss, more beautiful skin, better condition, deeper sleep and less time spend in the bed with easier wake-up, awakened and stronger sexuality. While making it possible to release body toxins, this method is then an invaluable help in the weaning of the medicinal dependences, from tobacco and alcohol in particular. Besides its toxin and fat elimination action, this Detox Bath's or packing's potency resides in the fact that:
1. It works on the groin area, one of the highest nerve-concentration areas in the body, hence its positive effect on mood, sleep and energy.
2. The groin houses main arteries, so the bath or packing greatly improves blood circulation and digestion.
3. It stimulates the root chakra, which governs sexual energy and reproductive organs. It helps regulate the menstrual cycle, and has been used by Louis Kuhne to treat impotence. It is also beneficial for low libido and menopausal symptoms. Regularity and repetition is key, evaluate after 60 days.

(*) Tight clothing or underwear, not to speak about synthetic as woman's panties (all modern practices unknown by our ancestors), around the abdomen and pubic area increases body temperature and static electricity-stress from accumulated electro charges. Avoid wearing tight pants, pantyhose, swimming suits, biking shorts or leotards for long periods. Cotton allows your genital area to "breathe." Don't wear underpants at night. Stay clothes-free whenever possible. Understand the differences between 'textiles', 'nudists' and naturists' and enjoy the latter. For more details on Kuhne 'pureinsideout.com' or on naturism 'naturistsociety.com', 'britishnaturism.org' or 'inf-fni.org'.

What are some signs that detoxification is necessary?
"Foggy brain", poor sleep habits, irritability, hormonal disorders, skin problems, weight gain, food allergies or intolerances, frequent colds, headaches, inflammation, constipation.

Watch your stool
Too hard? Too slow? Once every 3 days?
Once a day is a minimum, three times or 'one per meal' is better.

"The whole point of good digestive health is to reduce bite-size chunks to absorbable molecules: via mechanical chewing in the mouth, via cleaving by acids and one enzyme in the stomach, via cleaving by huge numbers of enzymes in the small intestine and to a much lesser degree in the large intestine."
~ Han van de Braak *BSc LicAc MCSP SRP MBAcC.*

Avoid refined food products like white bread, white rice, pastries, pasta's,.... Instead add extra fibers (25 gram a day) to your salads, pastas, soups, mashed potatoes, ..., but always with extra liquid before or after please! Try whole meal flour bread products and whole grain bread with leaven not yeast. Try an old fashioned German 'black' wheat bread. That is how our ancestor made it for centuries. Yeast and bleached white flour pastries are food industry gadgets for spoiled and lazy to chew consumers.
'Fruit and vegetables never enough!'
Drink minimum 8 glasses of water a day. Preferably with low mineral content (less than 100 mg/l TDS) and always without chlorine or fluoride, of course!
Use daily either yoghourt, kefir, sauerkraut or other fermented products like miso or tempeh to improve or balance your bowel bacteria with these 'good' bacteria or 'Probiotic' bacterial cultures. These products are easy to digest, fight diarrhea and help to strengthen our immune system.
Fibers, bran like oat bran is loaded with soluble fiber, which is sticky and combines with water to form a thick gel which helps greatly with your bowel movement and reduces the transit time.

On top researchers have reported that oat bran helps reduce blood cholesterol levels.

Color? Your stools should be dark brown. If they are pale brown, gray, yellow or dry and hard, your bile is low and your liver, meaning you, is in trouble.

Start-Up or Spring cleaning: tribal communities were familiar with annual periods of starvation and survival. Most religions include it in their rules.

You too can have your good reasons to step back for some days or weeks and have some self-starvation. Set your target-Measure up-Buy the needed good stuff-Program & find the TIME-Be courageous- Start the healing regime. Always start first day with drinking digestive and **liver cleaning** herbal infusions and best a rectal colon cleaning. Always drink pure water with low mineral content (less than 100mg/l preferably) like 1 liter per 30 kilo of bodyweight spread equally over the day. Infusing the body with pure water will immediately stimulate your kidneys, liver and digestive systems functions. It will boost your metabolism, which in turn accelerates toxin and fat elimination.

Get a ready from the shelf bowel movement supplement or your own mixture from the herborist based on herbs as senna leaves and pods, cascara sagrada aged bark, and cape aloe leaf. Take it in the evening and contractions will start within 6 to 8 hours. Once your bowel function is normal again you can continue the following weeks with a cleaning supplement like a prepared and sound Detox mixture (try 'methoddraine.com') add it to your first 1.5 liter of pure water and drink it throughout the day. Or get again your own mixture from the pharmacist based on clay powder (see also next page), apple fruit pectin, freshly ground flax seed, slippery elm bark, cinnamon powder, fennel seed, marshmallow root, and acid washed activated charcoal. Mix a table spoon in pure water or juice and drink 5 times a day. These combinations will draw out poisons, toxins, heavy metals like lead, cadmium and mercury, even radioactive materials like strontium-90, any known or unknown chemical and pharmaceutical-drug residues ever swallowed. Once your thorough bowel cleaning is ongoing you can add a supportive colonic hydrotherapy or irrigation.

If you need some motivation watch the video of Dr. Shinya Hiromi: 'dr-hiromi-shinya-colon-therapy' and 'mynht.com' and remember that in the United States, colorectal cancer is the second leading cause of death.

Colon cleaning if unknown to you consider for starters a thorough 'colonics' to remove waste from the large intestine in a natural way with the help of pure water under hygienic conditions. Simultaneous abdominal massages, will have a dislodging effect of colonic deposits. Colonic irrigation is an internal bathing and workout of the colon. Enemas involve the introduction of water into the colon through the rectum. It is the first and most effective detoxification the body can experience as you are literally washing out the body's main waste disposal unit. When the body suffers with chronic constipation, disease, yeast overgrowth (Candida), irritable bowel syndrome (IBS), and diarrhea there can be re-absorption into the blood stream of toxins that should have emptied via the bowel. This is known as autointoxication or leaky gut. The consequence of this is that the other eliminative organs of the body have to deal with more toxins than necessary and can suffer too. Any conditions related to the kidneys, skin, lungs and lymphatic system can have their origins in a congested colon. The benefits of   colonic irrigation can often be quickly observed in the form of improved bowel function together with clearer skin, more mental clarity and fewer headaches. Circulatory, immune, inflammatory and weight problems can also often improve with colonic treatments when accompanied by recommended eating and lifestyle changes. Athletes have opted for colon therapy to improve metabolic efficiency. Repeat the above 'Detox' program after 6 at latest 12 months. Get professional help at: 'cchcc.ca'

Drugs and herbs can have different effects on different people and should be taken in consultation with a good naturopath or doctor. Anyone considering a detox diet should consult a qualified health professional and/or their medical doctor first.

Worms, parasites? Lots of garlic is great for expelling worms, whether eaten or used in enemas and combined with black walnut inner hulls. You can also add pumpkin seeds to your salads. Or get professional advice.

Liver cleaning: deep breathing flushes the liver, eating smaller portions but +5 times a day just as fasting helps the liver. Our 'Garladior' is a continuous cleaner of your liver otherwise have a thorough liver and gall bladder cleaning with an own made blender mixture of 8 ounce/225 gram apple or citrus juice (add the peel if organic), same amount of pure water, a nice clove of garlic or two and a similar chunk of ginger. Optionally, certainly if you have them fresh available, you can add any bitter herb, root or leaves like from dandelions, artichoke, chicory, milk thistle or parsley.

Blood cleaning: there are many fine 'detox' teas and herb mixtures available on the market, but find one with or add yourself curcuma; burdock leaf is a strong blood purifier as nettle leaf, red clover and yellow dock root (*).

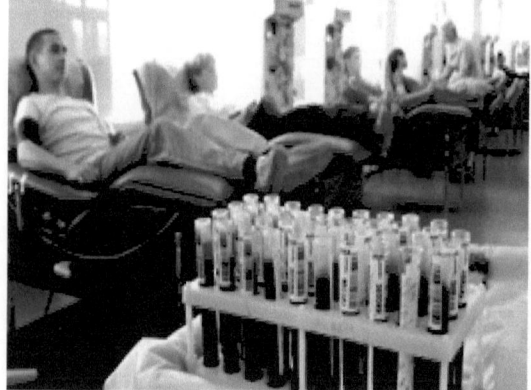

Nanotechnology will soon allow people to have their blood plasma cleaned relatively inexpensively says Leonid Melamed, the head of Russia's Nanotechnology Corporation. He added that fitness centers and beauty parlors could soon use nanotechnology to offer 'plasmopheresis' to their customers.

(*)This herb (*Rumex crispus*) can also stimulate a bowel movement within a few hours after ingestion to help remove lingering waste from your intestinal tract.

Efficient elimination can help prevent toxins from getting into your liver, gallbladder and bloodstream and this decreases the workload on these systems.

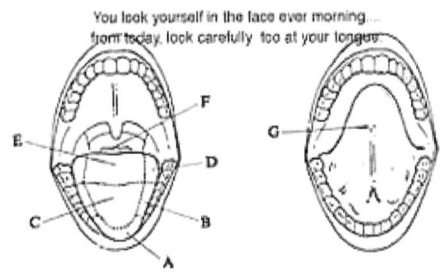

Natural Oil blood and general detox: a tablespoon of cold pressed sunflower, sesame oil, olive or cod liver oil (with lemon taste if you prefer) pulled in the top back of your mouth, chewed on and swished, chomped and squeezed through the teeth for +10 minutes at first in the morning will clean your tongue and throat area from mucus and possibly even detox your blood by help of your mouth enzymes. Spit the milky end result out in the toilet, never swallow, as unhealthy and clean your mouth. Finish by drinking 2 glasses of pure water. Repeat daily and evaluate after +30 days (*). During the oil-pulling and swishing process your metabolism is intensified, which will lead to improved health. Watch the possible improvement on gums, teeth color, a relaxed feeling on waking up, disappearing dark pouches below the eyes, anew appetite and energy, better memory and deep sleep. Indeed is the Ayurveda learning us about tongue diagnosis and does your tongue accurately reflects the state of your digestive system- from rectum to esophagus, including the stomach, small intestines, colon (large intestine), pancreas, spleen, liver and gall bladder. Read more 'hps-online.com/ntongue'.
(*) Give it and other natural treatments a month for every year you had the problem you are curing. The intention is not to prevent you from dying, but at helping you to live.

Algae Detox: Sea vegetables classified as brown algae, including arame, hijiki, kombu (kelp) and wakame (nori), have been shown to cleanse the body of toxic pollutants. They also have fat burning properties. You can get extra related information 'seaweedireland.com'.

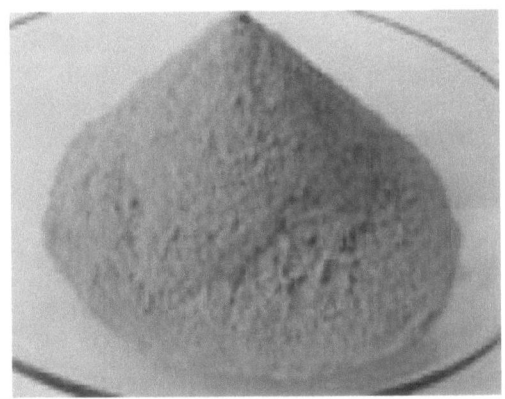

Clay Detox: white, green or brown clay, 'healing earth' or loess-powder, taken internally does kill bad bacteria in the gut. Clay may help fight drug-resistant germs. ``Since people existed, they have used clays for medicinal purposes," said Lynda Williams, a research professor at Arizona State University, in Tempe. Used internally as a gastrointestinal therapeutic product it acts as a cleansing sponge in absorbing impurities, such as gastric acid, gases, bacteria, excess fats and toxic materials, from the gastro-intestinal (GI) system. Ultra fine clay normalizes microbial flora in the intestine and prevents constipation. Half to one teaspoon in a glass of water two times a day (morning and evening) will do. *Not to combine with pharmaceutical medicines, consult your doctor.*

Fasting: If not 40 days, as found in many religions, +7days starvation will do ½ the miracles and even 1 full day, your Sabbath, might clear your mind, as there it all starts, and be a start of a new you. Any fast longer than 48 hours should be medically supervised, consult your physician.

Anyhow **re-start** after any Detox-cure the healthy way with slowly and moderately re-introducing to your plate fruits, vegetables, nuts, balanced foods preferably raw, juiced, fermented or steamed, pro-biotics and plenty of 'mineral-low' drinking water.

Get totally re-balanced with the Lesik™ 'ferments of life' cure: these unique, cellular balancing, pro-biotic food supplements ensure a good performance of the cellular breathing and scoring of the clogged cells, enabling the body to work properly and on its own.

After **ten years of use** on very diverse cases, the following can be confirmed as possible effects of this 'Probiotics' cocktail holding an enormous concentration of bio-available **free electrons**:
Biological Regulator (in particular of the intestinal functions: constipation/diarrhea).
- Regulator of weight. - Regenerator and anti-ageing. -
Anti-infectious and antiviral.
- - Stimulating immunizing defenses. - Attenuator of the side effects of chemical drugs.
Read and learn more: 'fermentsoflife.com'.

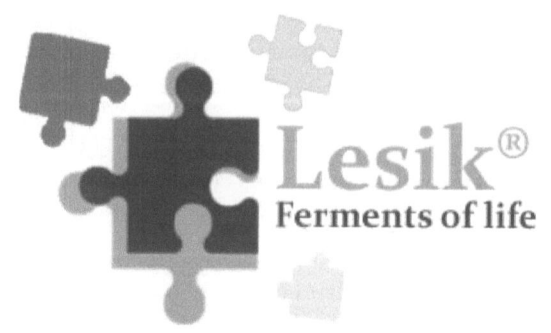

"Here a single product in its kind which corrects the 'terrain' while acting on all the cells of the body, repairs the small intestine, which stops the penetration of toxins in the body and allowing a much better assimilation of the vitamins and minerals." ~Yves Gillard M.D.

"In serious pathologies, the progressive clogging of the membranes reaches the stage of blocking, here only these products resulting from very strict and specific fermentation can restore an exchange flow, starting elimination reactions and later a return to the standards."
~Doctor Jeanne Rousseau, former president of BE-Association, born 1915.

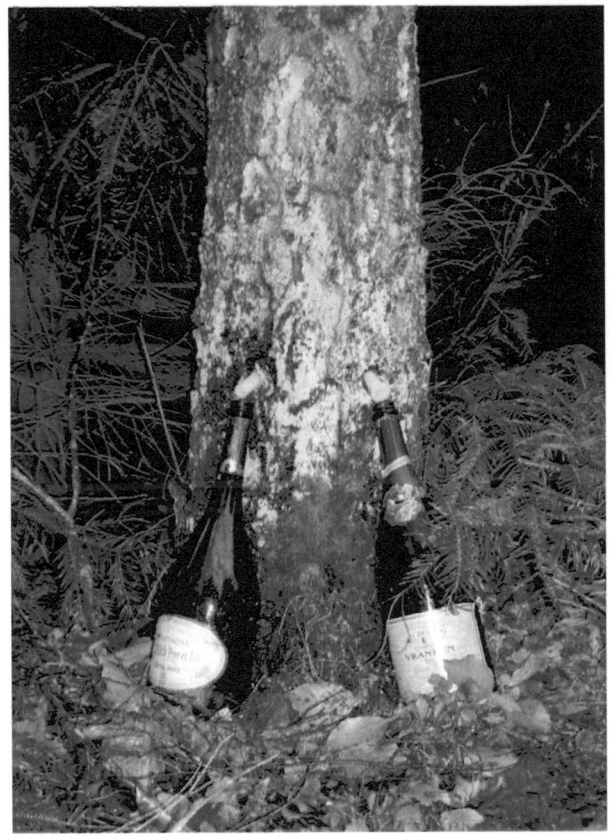

Silver-birch juice: The healing properties of the birch are known from time immemorial. Drinking twice a day a cup of freshly collected birch juice, in the spring when the tree wakes up from its winter sleep, is a true rejuvenation cure, an elixir. The juice contains natural glucose and fructose, mineral salts, oligo-elements and vitamin C and vitamins of the B-group. It is a strong diuretic (kidney cleaner), maintains or restores vitality after winter, lowers the levels of toxic substances in metabolism, clears skin and cleans the blood. If you cannot find the real thing then make your own 'juicy-infusion' from fresh birch leaves.

Sun therapy: Sunlight has an extremely positive effect on the human body, leading to the vital production of vitamin D which strengthens bones and increases resistance to disease and acts as a stimulator of the self healing ability of the body.

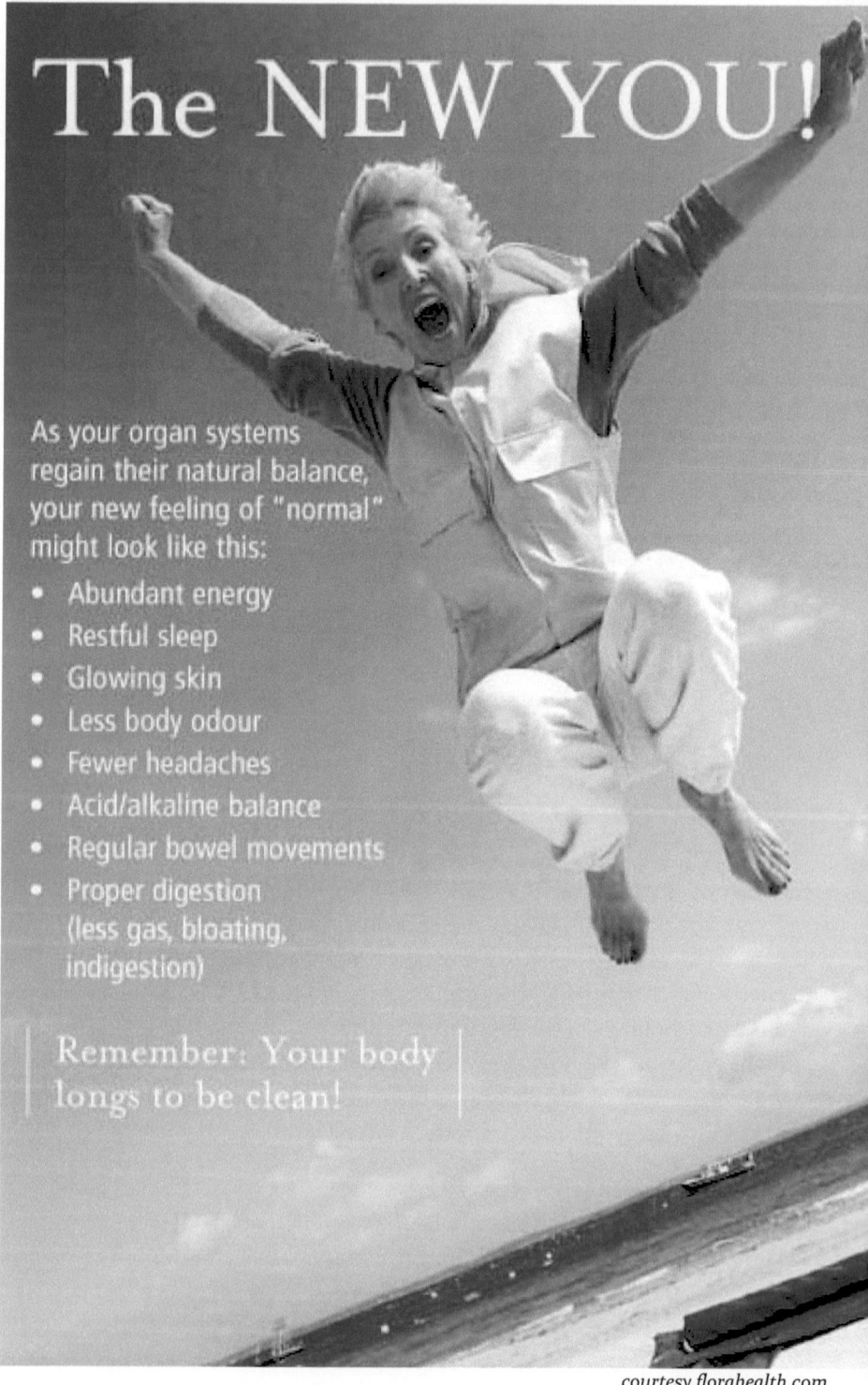

courtesy florahealth.com

Light and Color-therapy:
Colors not only co-define our look but also help to define our moods and are therefore important in generating a feeling of well being.

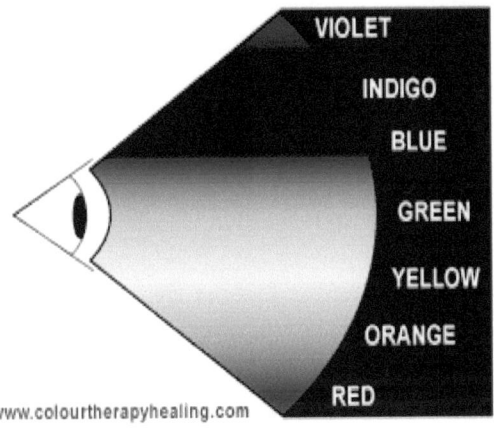

Violet: promotes awareness and consciousness
Blue: brings peace and quietness when sleep disturbances or anxieties are involved.
Green: is a calming, relaxing color helping to balance the mind.
Yellow/Orange: symbolizes joy and happiness. It helps raise one's spirit and enhances creativity.
Red: revitalizes, improves circulation and maximizes calorie burning.

Each color has a different wavelength and frequency. The color RED has a frequency of around 430 trillion vibrations a second. A high frequency light wave, as violet, has a higher **energy** than that of a low frequency light wave, as red for instance.

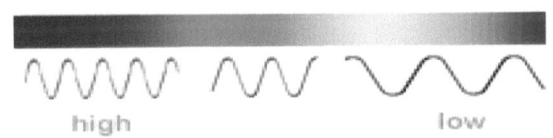

Air-therapy: starts with a zero-smoke tolerance! We can survive weeks without food, days without water, but only minutes without air thus oxygen. As mentioned earlier because of shallow breathing habits we can deny ourselves optimal levels of oxygen for better health. So use 'stomach' breathing!
air ionization: negative ions are lost as they adhere to walls, fabric materials, air-conditioning ducts, tobacco smoke, smog and crowds of people. Electrically charged aerosol particles (large air-ions) and electrostatic fields cause pollutants to settle on human skin. Moreover, air concentration of natural small air-ions, favorable for humans, is limited in city and many indoor environments. Radiation from space, air, rocks, and even some soils adds negative ions back into the air, as do sunshine, living green trees, and the breakup of water droplets, as occurs around waterfalls and the ocean surf. The earth's most tranquil and refreshing regions are thus loaded with billions of negative ions. Air near waterfalls, mountains, beaches and forests are among those places where ionization levels are in complete and

natural balance. After a lightning storm, most of us feel invigorated and refreshed. This is because the electrical storm has generated trillions of tranquilizing negative ions that ease tension and leave us full of energy. So get you first 'cup of air' in true nature!

Combine by going outside in the fresh air and take 1~10 slow, deep, abdominal breaths after each meal (helps digestion by massaging) and just before retiring for the night.

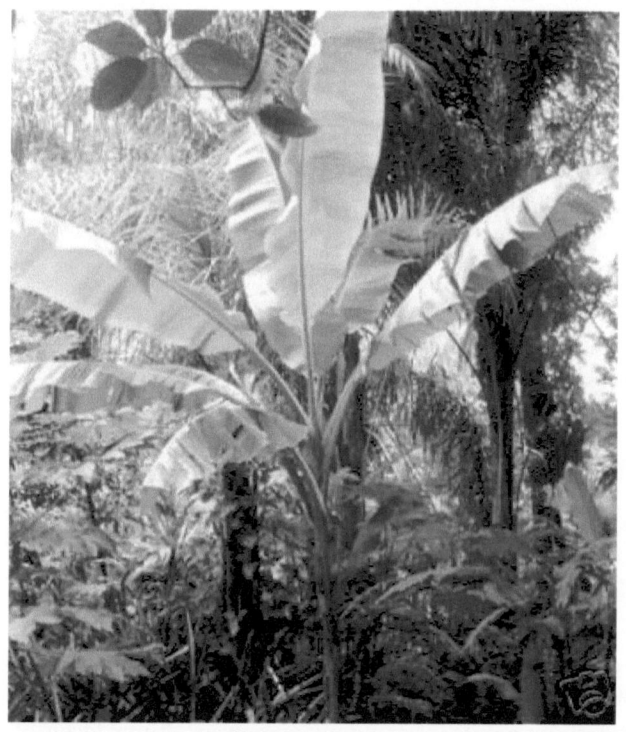

Only a handful of studies have investigated the use of vegetation as a means of removing or reducing levels of airborne microorganisms. This has sometimes been referred to as "growing clean air." Several common house plants are believed to help clean the air in our homes and offices by removing trapped chemical vapors (formaldehyde, benzene, TCE), carbon monoxide. Here a short list of them: rubber plant or ficus, aloe vera, fig trees, spider plant, Dracaena(corn plant), English ivy (hedera), Boston fern, Spathiphyllum (peace lily), Schefflera (umbrella tree), and elephant ear philodendron. VOG's (organic chemicals) can be absorbed best by the **banana tree**. Change your living room in a purifying 'rimbou'!

Ionizers enhance the environment with healthy negative ions. The overall effects of air ionization will depend on the individual person. There are some physicians prescribing air ionization for use in combating allergies like hay-fever & sinusitis, asthma symptoms and fatigue. **Negative air ionization therapy** is an experimental non-pharmaceutical treatment for seasonal affective disorder (SAD) and mild depression. "Negative air ionization has the potential to reduce the concentration of airborne microorganisms." ~ PennState Dept. of Architectural engineering.

Music Therapy: music influences positively on body and mind. The right choice of music for relaxation and meditation can make us cheerful, more balanced and reduce stress. Music listening can relax your stiffen muscles and decrease the stress. Endorphins and serotonins can be raised by music too and as such reduce pain and depression. Music having affirming lyrics will fill your brain with positive thoughts.

Steambath: The skin is the largest organ in the body and, through the pores it plays a major role in the detoxifying process. Most cultures around the world have their own versions of the sweat bath including the Turkish with their 'hamam'. A typical steam bath has a temperature of maximum 50C with a humidity of 100%. The mayor benefits of sweat bathing are the waste and toxins elimination action through the pores. Other sweat bath benefits include improved circulation, weight and fat loss, skin cleansing and body and mind relaxation.

Infrared (IR) cabin: as the body temperature rises by infrared heat perspiration occurs and blood circulation increases. The muscles and organs are stimulated and toxic waste is removed from your body while enjoying a pleasant cabin temp. of ~48C. Used by medical professionals for sports injuries and Detox. Speeds up metabolic processes of vital organs and glands, including endocrine glands. In an IR cabine you produce not only more sweat than in a traditional sauna, but important **only 80 to 85% of the sweat is wate**r with the non-water portion being principally cholesterol, fat-soluble toxins, toxic heavy metals, sulfuric acid, sodium, ammonia and uric acid. 30 minutes sessions.

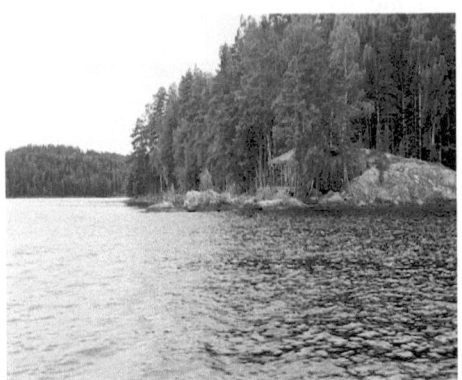 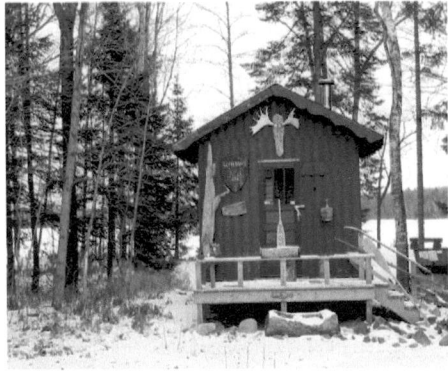

Sauna thousand or more years of history: using sauna for detoxification purposes is an ancient tradition practiced by different cultures around the world; the Finnish or Swedish sauna, the Russian banya, the Native American sweat lodge or inipi, the Turkish hamam, even the Japanese onsen. The skin is our largest organ and sweating is one of the body's most important 'detoxification' pathways. Similar advantages as IR cabin but less pronounced as 95% of sweat is water, cabin temperature 85-95C. One usually goes to the heat only for periods of six to twelve minutes at a time, maybe four times altogether, with in between similar period to cool down in the air or while swimming or having a short cold shower, or a snow-roll.

!**Check with your physician.** If you do not feel comfortable in a sauna, maybe you should do without it. This information is provided for educational purposes only. Consult your own physician regarding the applicability of any opinions or recommendations with respect to your symptoms or medical condition.

How to use diaphragm breathing!

When the metabolic process occurs in your body, oxygen is one of the vital components for this reaction to take place. By being properly oxygenated, you keep your body's oxygen levels high and your metabolism stays at an optimum level.

When you exercise, for instance, you increase your body oxygen intake and consequently you increase your metabolism. Most of us have become accustomed to shallow breathing (using online the top $1/3^{rd}$ of the lungs), but by deliberately breathing properly you can oxygenate your system. Proper breathing (also called stomach or abdominal breathing) happens in the lower area of your lungs where your oxygen capacity is highest. A deep breath should be in your **diaphragm** – just watch a sleeping baby breath and you will know how natural breathing occurs.

Deliberate breathing is a highly effective natural metabolism booster. Here is a simple breathing technique that will help you raise your metabolism:
You should breathe in the following ratio 1:4:2 (Inhale through your nose exhale through your mouth.)
Inhale for 1 count, hold for 4 counts and then exhale for 2 counts.
If you inhale for 3 seconds, you would hold for 12 seconds and exhale for 6 seconds.

You exhale thus twice as long as you inhale because that is when you eliminate toxins from your body via the lymphatic system. When you hold you can fully oxygenate your system and allow oxygen exchange.

Doing this type of exercises, on daily basis and minimum 21 days in a row, will enable you to switch step by step and automatically from shallow upper chest breathing (as by +90% of western people)to a normal full long breathing. The breath pace will then be slower but deeper. All the benefits will be yours.
Yogi learn the full breathing which always starts with abdominal breathing and continue with the thoracic (breast) and clavicular (upper lung) breathings.

Need **motivation**? Learn about the real figures: 'taichibreathing.com'.

Action: You must take at least 10 deep breaths a minimum of 3 times a day! It will take less than 3 minutes and you will feel a surge of energy go through your body.
Do it well: on average you breathe 23.000 times a day. You can double to quintuple your oxygen intake while breathing only 13.000 times a day!

The truth is present in every culture since ages. In relation to breathing we talked already about the Chinese approach with Qigong, but there are also the Indian yoga breathing techniques as with the **Pranayama**'s. For some visualizations look the video's at 'youtube.com/watch?v=mvdiMjSgItg&NR=1' or 'youtube.com/watch?v=t7WFq17NxWA&NR=1' and maybe first to understand better about the mayor increase of lung capacity with correct diaphragmatic breathing, about improving the sound of your voice, improving of your comfort feeling, peak performance and much more 'youtube.com/watch?v=23ctmPTwgGY&NR=1'.

Extra motivation: By adjusting the speed and depth of breathing, the brain and lungs are able to regulate the blood pH minute by minute. The amount of carbon dioxide (a waste product of the metabolism of oxygen, which all cells need) exhaled, and consequently the pH of the blood, increases as breathing becomes faster and/or **deeper**.

Smoking: NO comments!
Fanatic or addicted smoking is a slow suicide. Smokers fall for the aggressive marketing of the big cigarette brands. Yes, you can stop this risky behavior. It starts in your mind. "When I stop smoking I gain weight". Well not any more if you follow the "**EnjoyVity**" path. Getting or preserving a clean body and mind as talked about in these chapters will definitely make you quit.

Remember smoking will on average cost you **6 years** of your life not to speak of the medical cost and the stress involved once getting sick of it for yourself and your beloved ones. Stop fooling yourself.

About our body of cells and energy: our almost 600 quintillion (*) body cells operate electrically. In fact, our cells are an "electromagnetic resonator" capable of emitting and absorbing radiations of every frequency. GEORGE LAKHOVSKY in 1930: "each living being is simultaneously an emitter and receptor of electromagnetic radiation."
(*)*There are also roughly 600 quintillion atoms in just a drop of water.*

Each cell has 1.17 volts of electrical power. That means you have about 900 quintillion volts of energy contained within your physical body right now.

"The cell is immortal. It is merely the fluid in which it floats that degenerates. Renew this fluid at intervals, give the cells what they require for nutrition, and the pulsation of life may go on forever." ~Dr. Alexis Carrel, Nobel Prize winner

Put simply, all of your body functions rely on the electrical energy released from the unity of the 'charge' of the molecules in it and the opposite 'charge' in food water or air that enters it. ~Dr. Robert Young

Why do we rave on so much about **negative ions**? Because the result of every move we make (a net spending of electrical energy) is a positively charged body.

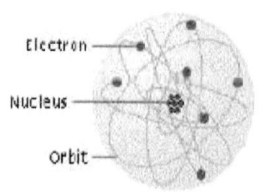

The molecules in your body are left holding a positive charge. They are unavailable for future 'couplings' unless we get a new batch, of attractive and giving negative ions, in quickly.

Cells are made of molecules and these of atoms. Atoms are the smallest pieces of an element that keep its chemical properties. Although you still look the same, we hope, as a year ago **98% of your atoms** are renewed through the air you breathe, the food you eat and the water you drink. Here today, completely gone in some years, renewed down to the last single atom, we endure only in the shape, form and pattern that are assured by our genetic blueprint.

"**Your body is younger than you think**", states Dr. Frisen, a stem cell biologist at the Karolinska Institute in Stockholm " he has also discovered a fact that explains why people behave their birth age, not the physical age of their cells: a few of the body's cell types endure from birth to death without renewal, and this special minority includes some or all of the cells of the cerebral cortex."

An average person takes in 1.5 ton of matter every year as food, drinks and oxygen. All this matter has to learn to be you. Every year! New atoms will have to learn to remember your childhood. ~ Tor Norretranders

Nataraj - the cosmic dancer - represents the constant **biodance of life**-creation, maintenance and transformation and indicates the perfect balance between life and death. Shiva's dance is the most inspiring and pragmatic act typifying the eternal rhythm which is the cause of the infinite creative process. Shiva is the presiding deity of the mind. The entire universe created by Shiva is his SHAKTI (Prakriti, or Nature) or **energy**. Shiva's dance movements represent the movement of his SHAKTI or energy. ~ 'hinduism.co.za'.

An atom is formed by a positive nucleus and around **negatively charged electrons**. Hydrogen is the smallest atom. Electrons can behave as waves. An electron in atomic orbit is in resonance. The mass of the electron is 9.10 x 10^{-28} grams. For comparison, a U.S. penny has a mass of 2.5 grams; so, 2.7 x 10^{27} or 2.7 billion billion billion electrons would weigh as much as a penny! We are now in the field of quantum mechanics, the science of the very small.

The picture of this **M-51 galaxy**, shows two different swirls connected by two energetic paths which is a completely independent wave (Quantum) formation and the **Hydrogen atom** resembles this design . Or in Einstein's wording: "Small atom and large galaxies formations must have the' same behavior." Further "The Hydrogen Atom is the basic smallest, stable unclosed quantum, wave- particle formation" and "The brain is a perfect gravitational wave."
~ Dr. Tejman Chaim

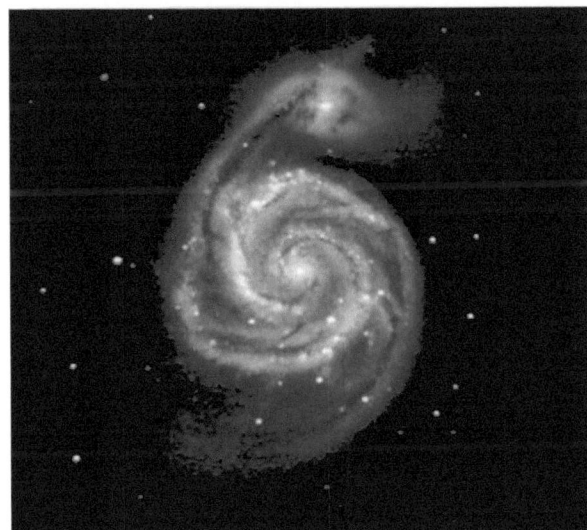

From the **macro-cosmos** of our universe and galaxy to the **micro-cosmos** of our cell atoms or DNA it's all about electro-magnetism. Look also at these "YinYang" painting and 3D animation and rethink this part of the chapter: 'youtube.com/watch?v=6R8tEtE2naI&hl=fr' and
'youtube.com/watch?v=SRmmJqaJA98&feature=related'

"When we consider organic life in the light of biophysics, we find that electrical phenomena are at the root of all cellular life and we conclude that the end of everything is an electrical charge." ~ Dr J. Belot

Researchers have found that the (to them) previously unknown electric fields inside of cells are as strong, or stronger, as those produced in lightning bolts. Previously, it has only been possible to measure electric fields across cell membranes, not within the main bulk of cells, so scientists didn't even know cells had an internal electric field. University of Michigan researchers led by chemistry professor

Raoul Kopelman found electric fields as strong as **15 million volts** per meter, up to five times stronger than the field found in a lightning bolt.

Professor L.C.Vincent calculated already in 1976 that every human spermatozoid got 350 x more electrons than the ovule, creating a lightning bolt discharge of **480.000 Volt** as fecundation thus conception takes place. L.C. Vincent is the inventor of the **Bio-Electronic Terrain** (substrate) **Analysis** of the body and other fluids and this since 1935. This BEV-science measures the electro magnetism of our micro-cosmos. .Professor Vincent once correctly said: "Withdraw the substrate from the illness, and the illness will starve to death!" (read also in chapter 6)

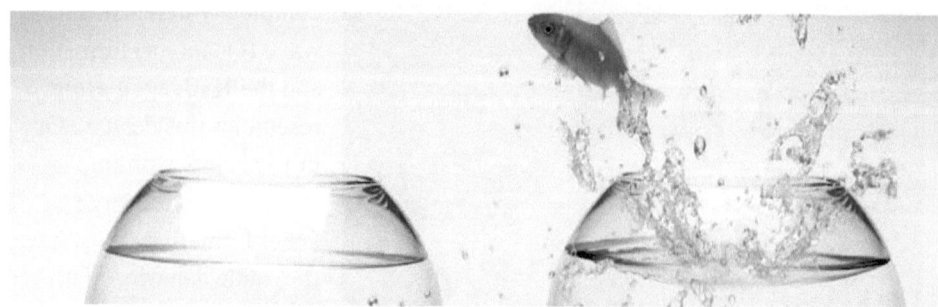

If you feel like this unhappy fish **change your 'Terrain'!**

There is no difference between 'Chi' or ' Prana' and 'bio-electric ' energy. Yin equals passive and Yang equals aggressive energy. When your body is in a balance state the **energy flows** freely through the **meridians**, pathways of the energy, and you are free of illness and calm.

What is oxidative stress? It's a large rise (becoming less negative) in the cellular reduction potential also called **redox** potential, oxidation/ reduction potential or **ORP**. Oxidative stress is involved in many diseases, such as cancer, Alzheimer, heart failure and chronic fatigue syndrome, but it may also have an impact on your body's aging process. The destructive aspect of oxidative stress is the production of free radicals and peroxides. **Free radicals, or** ROS, being the "reactive oxygen species" interact with other molecules within cells. This can cause oxidative damage, auto-oxidation, to proteins, membranes and genes. More overall stress, environmental pollution and less quality in our diets, mean that we are exposed to more free radicals than ever before. Antioxidants (see also page 46) will neutralize the free radicals. Fresh fruit and vegetables should be your first and abundant source of antioxidants. The healthy relationship between oxidants (like free radicals) and the reducers (like antioxidants) of the body is thus called the **Red-Ox** balance, a basic condition of health. Meaning an **overdose** of antioxidants will lead also to a weak immune system. Eating and drinking with moderation and variation will respect this **balance**, over-supplementing may not.

If the mechanisms of regulation are overflowed beyond the bearable variations (**homeostasis**) the 'Terrain' (substrate) becomes oxidized (positive electricity) or reduced (negative electricity), it cannot function any longer normally and produces corresponding pathologies (cardiovascular, autoimmune, infectious, cancers, osteoporosis, Alzheimer...). The in this chapter and book described cleaning procedures and habits will bring or keep your body in balance.

Dr. Fritz Popp, a European working with fellow scientists from Princeton stated, "The DNA molecule transmits its blueprint information to other cells by means of an encoded burst of coherent ultra-violet **laser light**." (read also next chapter)

Einstein received his Nobel Prize for his findings, that all waves have a dual quality: they are both wave like and particle like. The longer the wave length, the less particle-like it is. While long waves are extremely life supporting, short waves with high frequencies such as X-ray, Gamma waves, micro-waves etc. are dangerous and harmful.
Human beings are an open "radio system" made up of varying electromagnetic frequencies that naturally interact with all natural and man-made external energies. These energies play a large part in our health and well being.

Certain synthetic clothes are strong enough to set up a field that repels all negative ions in your immediate vicinity! Go stand on a mountain; it won't help much if you're wearing your favorite synthetic ski jacket or you walked there with synthetic panties or trousers on!

"Life is the dynamic equilibrium of all cells, the harmony of multiple radiations which react upon one another" and "The nucleus of a living cell may be compared to an electrical oscillating circuit. This nucleus consists of tubular filaments, chromosomes and mitochondria, made up of insulating material and filled with a conducting fluid containing all the mineral salts found in sea water."~ Georges Lakhovsky "Secrets of Live" a study on electromagnetic waves.
In other words, human body composed of ions, minerals and a high percentage of water, is a strong conductor of energy. Like metal, our body is a very effective antenna structure. When exposed to its natural frequency, human body will pick up or resonate with that frequency, resulting in good health.

Dr. Klinghardt teaches at his Academy of Neurobiology about the 5 levels of healing with at the second level the 'Energy Body' or 'body electric', with reference to Dr. Popp. It is the summation of all electric and magnetic events caused by the neuronal activity of the nervous system. www.klinghardtneurobiology.com/5LevelsColorMap.pdf

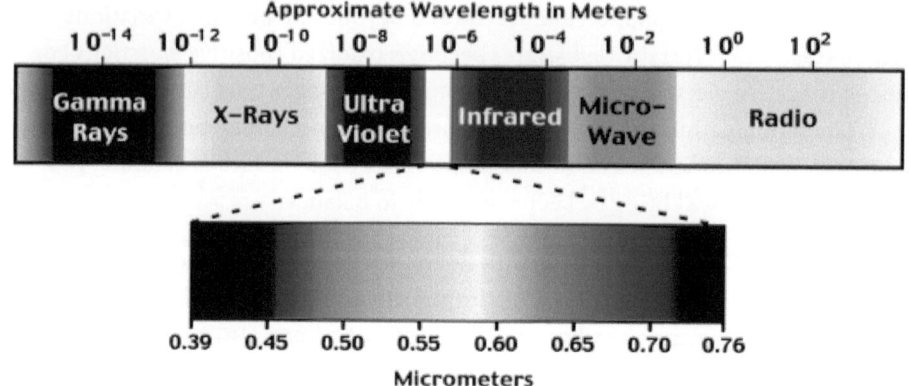

Various types of electromagnetic radiation as defined by wavelength. Visible light has a spectrum that ranges from 0.40 to 0.71 micrometers (μm). Source: 'PhysicalGeography.net'.

The dosimetry of exposure to radiofrequency (RF) electromagnetic (EM) fields of **mobile phones** is generally based on the 'specific absorption rate' (SAR, W kg^{-1}), which is the electromagnetic energy absorbed in the tissues per unit mass and time. The studying of electromagnetic wave interactions with the human body just start this century, don't ask for clear answers yet. 'Current electromagnetic (EM) safety guidelines for demonstrating compliance as well as some of the current measurement standards may well not be consistent with the basic restrictions and need to be revised.' ~Kuhn &Co IT IS Zurich 2009

On **'Bioresonance'** and the related therapy: toxic substances in the body can be eliminated just by erasing their pathological waves. Using the waves of substances, toxins and so on, for therapy, by reapplying the same waves but after reversing them, is the main and most important idea for healing in quantum medicine. And the waves - as we know - are one billion times more important than the substance. Frequencies from 10 Hz to 164 KHz are available in BRT. Our brain's frequency is 5 to 8 hertz, similar to the magnetic waves generated by the earth. 'dr-kessler.com'

Sorry if you wanted simply a **quick fix** without altering your actual lifestyle.

You really **want that change**? Then dare!
Change now for the better. Get a new 'Terrain'.

> **I believe the most important single thing, beyond discipline and creativity is daring to dare. ~Maya Angelou**

So remember say "No, thank you"
> to smoking

>> to superficial breathing

So remember you can add years to your life

> by detoxicating your body bi-annually

> by drinking minimum 8 glasses of water

> by cleaning and listening to your body

9. Have clear and clean thoughts

Worry and time have an inverse relationship. The more you have of one, the less you have of the other. Yet curiously both are suspended when you live in the now. ~Mike Dooley

Even in our today's 'flat world' the Babylon syndrome is still awake, we still think in boxes, the confusion of tongues(*) is omni-present. The gap between those of the West and the East remains huge. And what about North/South, American/Russian, politicians/citizens, fast food/slow food, rich/poor, carnivore/vegetarians, young/old, archer/crab, utopia/dystopia, Catholic/Muslim, bankers/savers, white/black, optimists/pessimists, burned-outs/bored-outs an ongoing list.
(*) over 30 different languages in Europe alone

Let's listen to the view and thundering voice of Winston Churchill:

"A pessimist sees the difficulty in every opportunity; an optimist sees the opportunity in every difficulty."

No fanatic-ism, maniacs-ism or perfection-ism so also NO overdone 'enjoyvity-ism'.

Stick with **positive** thinkers and winners. Similar as we asked earlier to create your 'healthy' network.

Do not argue with yourself. Think, decide and act.

Know that a healthy Mind contains a healthy Body …

If you think you're beaten, you are;
If you think you dare not, you don't;
If you'd like to win, but think, you can't
It's almost a cinch you won't.
If you think you will lose, you're lost;
For out in the world we find,
Success begins with a fellow's will,
It's all in the state of mind.
from 'The man who thinks he can'   ~Walter D. Wintle

Learn about the connection between 'Think' and 'Thank': 'tut.com'®

Respect the elderly, listen to their opinions, enjoy their calm, their way of keeping perspective, their   enriching stories which you might only understand and appreciate when they left you.
Respect is important because it helps build the inner strength which we believe is the key to achieving a long and healthy life.

"In the end, it's your mental attitude that's most important,"

"To develop a great mental game, it's critical to realize that your mental state affects the chemistry of your brain which in turn affects your ability to perform. Then, it's just a matter of reprogramming your mind to optimize your chemistry so you can play in the zone." ~ Michael Anthony

Over 80% of all cancers are caused by emotional and mental stress says dr Leonard Coldwell/*Instinct Based Medicine - How to survive your illness …and your doctor.*

Read mind setting books: John Naisbitt *Mindset*, Collins 2006
                               Carol Dweck *Mindset*, Random House 2007
                               Brault & Seaman *The Winning Mindset,* Center Line Press NY

Follow the 'inspirational': Robert Kiyosaki *Conspiracy of the Rich,* Hachette Book group NY, 2009 and   'conspiracyoftherich.com'

Learn 4+ languages, have 3+ hobbies, play 2+ instruments, love 1+ person

Never stop learning, reading, dialoging, contemplating, ascertaining,...

Think big and move forward with small steps

"A healthy diet is hardly the only prerequisite for a long life. Scientists say another key factor is your mind-set. That's to say, the emotional resources that enable you to cope with the stresses of daily life from missing the train to enduring the death of a loved one. Inner strength derives in part from vigorous activity, mental and physical."

Meditate, practice yoga, pray, bio-walk, relax your mind, breath consciously, ... and DAILY. Remember, also from John Lennon's 'beautiful boy', Emile Coué's mantra-like conscious autosuggestion: "Every day, in every way, it's getting better and better".

There is no need to and you cannot stop the time, but meditation will keep its importance in perspective

Understand well that time is always there for you and with you and in abundance.

Moving the body plays a key role in cleansing our bodies of garbage and scraps. It should not be used only when there is a problem with weight or to just build muscle mass. It should also be used to clear the mind, gain clarity, awareness and understanding. It is a perfect time to be alone with your thoughts so you can pray while involving yourself in an activity that you thoroughly enjoy. Moving your body should be effortless, exhilarating and meditative. From 'moving meditations': 'drstandley.com'

It is all about energy, wavelength and frequency (see also chapt. 8)

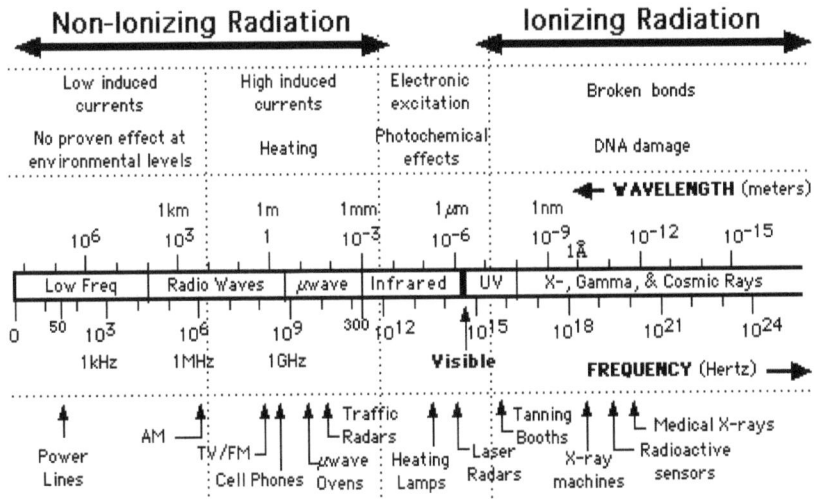

The bio frequency of a living healthy cell is 10 to the 13th Herz. The human body is a low energy irradiating source which can emit many kinds of physical frequencies ranging from infrared to weak microwave.

Extremely low-frequency magnetic fields (ELF-MFs) of 50 Hertz may already interfere with biological systems and facilitate oxidative damages in living cells.~ Fernanda Amicarelli & Co, Department of Basic and Applied Biology, University of L'Aquila, Italy.

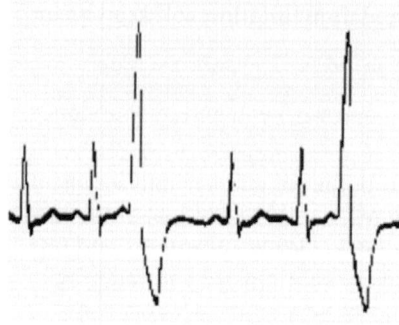

Undisputed evidence regarding the existence of electricity, thus energy, in the body are the electroencephalograph of the brain (EEG) and the electrocardiograph of the heart (EKG).

Mobile and WiFi: no panic but correct information is needed, while objective scientists sort things further out be reserved in its usage. For the moment we consumers could conclude that it is unwise and arguably dangerous to be exposed for long periods to the radiation from Wifi transmitters, cordless phones and mobile phones

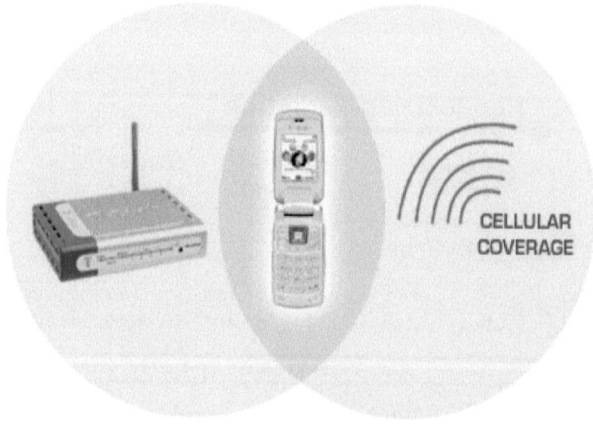

(especially their base stations, which run 24/7). So lets **keep it SHORT!** If the possible dangers and effects of electromagnetic exposure (on your fertility and even your off-spring) are of interest to you, which they should, then best read Andrew Goldsworthy BSc PhD, retired lecturer at the Imperial College Londondr., comments: 'hese-project.org/cell_phone_and_cell.pdf'

Extra on **electrosmog:** by 2011, New York will be the largest city in the world to use wireless water metering for water bills. Here some water parameters before and after 24 hour exposure to a mobile phone's electromagnetic field: pH 6.30/7.7, rH_2 (degree of oxidation) 27.5/33 and resistivity 28.000/1850. Just think and evaluate for yourself.

Energy-efficient lighting!? The 2002 WHO/IARC study confirmed already that economy light bulbs are possibly carcinogenic for humans.

Dr. Magda Havas Associate Professor, Environmental and Resource Studies Trent University, Peterborough, ON, Canada stated in her June 2008 study summary about Health Concerns associated with Energy Efficient Lighting and their Electromagnetic Emissions: "Alternative light bulbs (*LED*) are available that are much more energy efficient than CFL, do not contain mercury, do not produce radio frequencies or UV radiation, and do not make people sick."

Be it in French the message given by renown French scientific journalist Annie Lobe is clear: Economy light bulbs or compact fluorescent light bulbs (CFL's) create risky ELF's (magnetic fields of extreme low frequency), contain Hg (mercury) and give off radio frequencies (up to 200 Volt/meter) the latter makes them even illegal for sale.
Look at her visualizations and tests: 'tinyurl.com/ny7xdg' .

Further information on possible illnesses and effects of different kind of modern lighting devices by "Right to Light and Spectrum, Alliance for Light Sensitivity": 'tinyurl.com/lrzfet'.

So wait to exchange all your original incandescent light bulbs! Or at least be aware that the clean-up of *toxic* mercury bulbs if they break is a bit like a mini hazardous waste disposal program.

Last but not least, CFL's give limited spectrum lighting - which means that they only emit two rays of the seven rays emitted by the sun. Those of you who suffer from Seasonal Affective Disorder, need full spectrum lighting to counter the depressed mood that this affliction creates.

As least is that EHS or 'electro-hypersensitivity', also called radio wave sickness, is becoming the new treat or should we say epidemic as 35% of the population in developed countries has already many of the symptoms of EHS. The long list of symptoms includes neurological, cardiac, respiratory, dermatological, ophthalmologic and many other problems and pains.

Dr.Popp's biophoton energy (1970 University Marburg-Germany) is a photon of light emitted from a biological system and detected by biological probes as part of the general weak electromagnetic radiation of living biological cells. "Biophotonics" as science started with Erwin Schrödinger, Nobel prize Physics 1933:" the energy to do the work, to keep up life in the living matrix, comes from photons" and has been overtaken by the American National Science Foundation and established and developed in the mean time to one of the most forward looking fields of modern science and technology. Dr Popp: " tissue in pain is emitting less photons and dead cells don't emit photons." and on cancer development: "... one has to consider that by the lack of coherent electromagnetic energy the repair and communication system between cells gets damaged." More: 'ifescientists.de'.

It all starts in our mind!

What are brain waves? "Rhythmic fluctuations of voltage between parts of the brain resulting in the flow of an electric current, that has a pulsation frequency of 10 or more per second (>10Hertz)."

State	Frequency range	State of mind
Delta	0.5Hz - 4Hz	Deep sleep
Theta	4Hz - 8Hz	Drowsiness (also first stage of sleep)
Alpha	8Hz - 14Hz	Relaxed but alert
Beta	14Hz - 30Hz	Highly alert and focused

Delta waves are known for triggering the release of growth hormone, which provides healing, hence the reason why sleep is so important during the healing process.
The theta stage (4hz - 7Hz) has been found to increase learning capabilities.
The human brain is in the Alpha wave range between 8-12 Hz at its best to meditate or solve problems (Berger's waves). Learn more on brainwaves: 'taichibreathing.com'.

Train your brain: Brainwave 'entrainment', learns you to change your brain frequency towards the desired state, be it relaxation or enhanced attention. Brainwave generation is used in treatment of depression, low self-esteem, attention deficit disorder, weight control, drug and alcohol addiction and autism, to name a few. Learn more: 'bwgen.com'.

"The negative ion count per cubic centimeter at Yosemite Falls is over 100,000. On the other hand the count is far below 100 on the Los Angeles Freeways..." "Negative Ions promote alpha brain waves and increase brain wave amplitude, which translates to a higher awareness level." The metabolism is enhanced to create better utilization of nutrients from our foods and vitamins, while our brain's intuitive, nonlinear activities flow more smoothly. Jan Stolwijk, of the World Health Organization, stated that, "there is probably more damage done to human health by indoor air pollution than by outdoor pollution." Most people spend 70% to 80% of their time indoors! So improving the indoor air quality with the choice of sufficient and the right houseplants (read more on page 74)or a performing **air ionizer** (or **negative ion generator**) or airfilter is a must-do. Notebook producers ASUS have now started to include air ionizers in their computers. That not only helps clean the air around the user of allergens and germs, but also promotes airflow and circulation. Need more on air ionizers start here: 'ionlight.com' and 'surroundair.com'.

Water, air, and cleanliness are the chief articles in my pharmacopoeia. ~Napoleon I

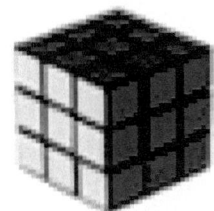

Oxygenate your brain.
Turn on your creativity exercises: play chess, keep a journal, read books, learn a language, play music, sing in choir or out loud in your bathroom, start a new 'fun' hobby, puzzle/Sudoku/crossword/quiz/..., ...

Educational Kinesiology (Edu-K)- enhanced learning through movement - was created by Dr. Paul E. Dennison and Gail E. Dennison through their extensive research in areas that include education, brain function, psychology, and applied kinesiology. Repatterning through brain gymnastics for children of all ages improves reading, learning and problem behaviors. Enjoy the Brain Gym ® movements in classrooms and businesses worldwide, as a tool to integrate the brain before learning, work, or sports activities, as well as during breaks: 'braingym.org'.

Stay in control of your emotions: doing focused, deep breathing relaxes the body and calms the mind, so combining this with your affirmations will make you more receptive to the positive suggestions, images, and feelings you are creating.

Stay emotionally and physically resilient.

EFT? 'Emotional Freedom Techniques' is an emotional, needle free version of acupuncture that is based on new discoveries regarding the connection between your body's subtle **energies**, your **emotions**, and your health, a natural healing aid you can use for almost everything. EFT has been able to **address the causes** of these energy disruptions with a gentle tapping procedure on head, torso and hands while using the fingertips.
Get your **free** introductions from Gary Craig himself: 'emofree.com'.
"Some day the medical profession will wake up and realize that unresolved emotional issues are the main cause of 85% of all illnesses. When they do, EFT will be one of their primary healing tools ... as it is for me." ~ Eric Robins, MD

Breath with your full lung capacity, step back, reflect, refresh, analyze, re-evaluate and re-oxygen.
A **MUST-DO** in these for many harsh times.

Practice your daily affirmation:

I AM ALWAYS TRUTHFUL, POSITIVE, AND HELPING OTHERS

as 'freely' served by Michael Anthony through his inspiring **'HappyBook'**, 'howtobehappy.org'.
A **MUST-READ**, to stop being afraid, to pump up your intelligence and happiness.

Alzheimer: to know that very soon in the US alone **10 million BabyBoomers** will get this ...disease! We are not going to let this happen, right.

Getting or being 65+ and concerned? Make the first 10 signs test: 'alz.org' for Europe start at 'alzheimer-europe.org' or 'dementia-in-europe.eu'.
a global figure for Europe for people with dementia over the age of 60 would be: **10.8 million** for 2020 and **15.9 million** for 2040.China and developing western Pacific will fast-grow towards +26 million people with dementia and the world total from 24 now to probably over 81 million. ~*Ferri, C.L. , Prince, M. et al. (2005), Global prevalence of dementia: a Delphi consensus study, The Lancet, Vol. 366, December 17/24/31, 2005.*

With such figures, epidemic becomes the right word, not disease.

The risk of developing Alzheimer's or vascular dementia appears to be increased by many conditions that damage the heart or blood vessels. These include high blood pressure, heart disease, stroke, diabetes and high cholesterol. Many of the **"EnjoyVity"** advices will protect from and correct or avoid most of these risks.

Amalgam! Toxic **mercury in tooth fillings** is one of the principal sources of oxidative stress (read page 120) on the organism of a great majority of people, increasing our need for 'more' antioxidant nutrients. Mercury also causes degeneration of brain neurons, as an educational film of the University of Calgary shows. 'movies.commons.ucalgary.ca '.

Lets focus on **PREVENTION**.

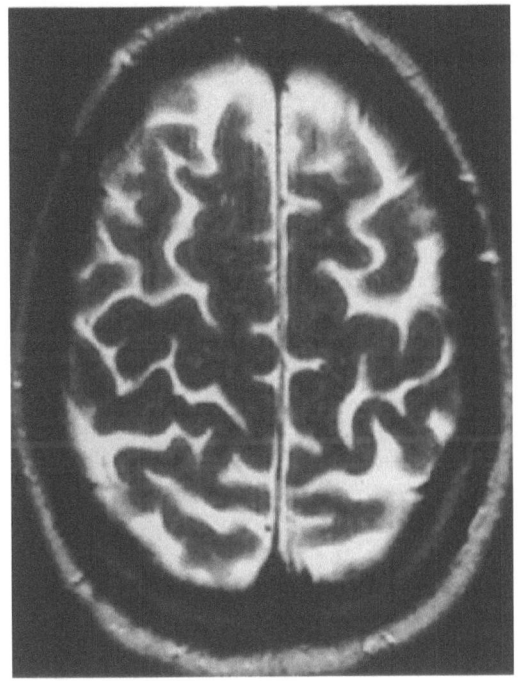

Outgoing people are 50 percent less likely to develop dementia, according to a recent study of more than 500 men and women age 78 and older from the Karolinska Institutet in Sweden. Participants also described themselves as not easily stressed.

Exercise brain and body, healthy thoughts and foods, get rid of overweight, manage your blood pressure, get enough sleep,... get or stay socially involved. Work to live and not vice versa. You start seeing the trees in the forest? Well yes, it is all inter-linked, as said earlier or later in this book. Everything in the human body is interconnected.

The more you **get in balance** the less you crave for sugar, carbohydrates, treated animal fat, alcohol, smoking,... and the better you can withstand fear, hastiness and stress.

Your prayer must be for a sound mind in a sound body.
Or from the original: 'orandum est ut sit *mens sana in corpore sano*' ~Juvenal

So remember say "No, thank you"
        to any -ism

        to fear and stress

So remember you can add years to your life

        by oxygenating your brain

        by getting and staying in balance

10. Know how and when to speak

"The gift of oratory wields a power more durable than that of a great king" ~W.Churchill

You are a human antenna, a transmitter so made to communicate and even without talking you are connecting with others.

Verbal communication transmits words and thoughts.
How good a speaker are you? Listen to your voice. Tape it.
Keep it subtle. It is about connection, seduction, respect, emotion and attraction.
Find out about intonation, frequency, warmth, speed, fluency, tremble, hesitations and pauses.

Often is 'not speaking' preferable. When you are silent you are also communicating!
If you want people's attention than you should build report, get and keep attraction.
Keep it flowing, liquid and soft.
Take care of your **feelings** through your unconscious **body language**. How you walk, move, stand, sit, have eye contact, gesticulate, mimicry or facial expression, touch ...and even misuse or abuse your mobile. To make the meaning of our words clear we use body language, it is a language without spoken words and is therefore called non verbal communication. A good speaker will pay attention to the body language signals from the audience and if possible adjust the speech 'delivering' accordingly.

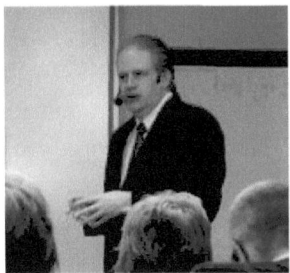

About the body language: learn from this basics table 'deltabravo.net' and from 'zanperrion.com' or an introductory video of **Zan Perrion** to start your transformation 'youtube.com/watch?v=nzezbYtLvtM&feature=channel'
by Mitchell Rose 'youtube.com/watch?v=x9YTxff3pHU' , but take care it is not that universal 'youtube.com/watch?v=Mi6h8zktO1s' . Check it out be-

fore travelling between continents. Learn from the best like **Kevin Hogan** 'kevinhogan.com/bodylanguage' and take his Free introduction with exercises about the basic components of communication 'kevinhogan.com/communication'

Many problems find auto-solutions if you let just time and silence work on it. Be thus at first a good listener.

People have mostly their answers 'al-ready' before they throw you the question. They just want confirmation, start a discussion or want to be polite before briefing you on their own more important life stories. Reply with an open question and you will learn from them the answer they were expecting from you, or at least the bulk of it.
Open questions create rapport, well, in case you listen to the answers. Observe.

Be empathic, curious and take things less personally.

Be prepared: learn about those you are going to meet, about their interests. Have a joke or anecdote ready.

Know your opening's sentence. Get visual aids if you are not confident.

The '20' principle: either during a phone call or during a meeting your first 20 words spoken, the first 20 seconds will set your opponent's mind as will the 20 centimeter (8") of your face you show. Even at the phone a smile on your open face can and will be felt at the other side of the line just as anxiety or dullness will; so for sure during a video-call you better show up with an open face. Read also under Chapter 7 about that **First Impression**.

To persuade someone it's not your words (7%) which prevail but your enthusiasm and the tone of your voice (38%) and even more important is your physical appearance as 55% of our communication is visual as shown in the studies by Albert Mehrabian/UCLA. People can thus see what you are not saying. If your body language doesn't match your words, you are wasting your time. Of course figures are never that 'absolute', but 'the how' you say it dominates and what you say is important.

If it is not in your genes, than build **your confidence** and learn the basic skills to phone and speak in public. It's all about practice, breathing, natural rhythm, the use of simple sentence structure and wording.

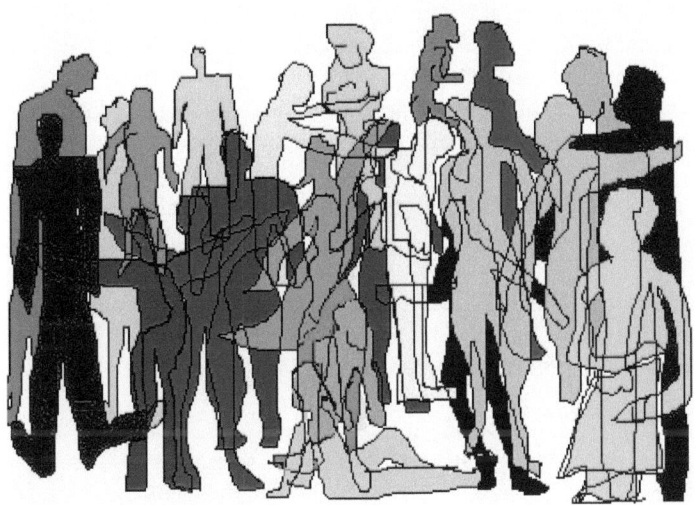

Enfolding Shadows

For your confidence and self-esteem **being lonely** for too long may not be a good thing. Ultimately we are all at some time alone, by ourselves, and ultimately lonely. To feel lonely is acknowledging that we are somehow fundamentally separated from each other, doomed to speak and yet never fully understood. It can feel like a cage or prison even while being surrounded by happy people. Loneliness can eat you away and can leave you suffering in silence.

Your OUTING. Step out! Learn to **love yourself**. Step out! Learn to help others. Speak out! Talk to yourself in your journal, in the mirror. Start with a smile to yourself then to others. Your positive approach will be rewarded, always. Share and learn more about loneliness 'webofloneliness.com'. Get some deep breaths and help yourself and the world while practicing the daily affirmation (details chapter 9):

**I
AM
ALWAYS
TRUTHFUL,
POSITIVE,
AND
HELPING
OTHERS**

Build your network: it is proven that having a strong network of friends, family and community is key to longevity. If you're happy and you know it, thank your friends—and their friends. But if you're sad, hold the blame. Researchers from Harvard Medical School and the University of California, San Diego have found that "happiness" is not the result solely of a cloistered journey filled with individually tailored self-help techniques. Happiness is also a collective phenomenon that spreads through networks like an emotional contagion.

Friends may help boost people's self-esteem. So connect, speak out and feel more confident.

Step away from your TV or PC screen and get out of your home.
Be socially active. In your neighborhood, your community, city or in the world ... Yes, be a cosmopolitan, as you know where you came from and the whole world is flat and yours.
Spread your positive message. **Dialogue!**

Go!
'myspace.com' with 254 million users or 'facebook.com' with 140 million users, 'tagged.com' 70 million and 'reunion.com' 51 million users.

Or what to say from 'ravelry.com' with 270.000 member lovers of knitting and crocheters, 'last.fm.com' 21 million music enthusiasts, but also 'imeem.com' 24 million searchers for music, video's and more 'italki.com' with 400.000 language freaks 'athlinks.com' for many fast bikers, 'badoo.com' 15 million, 'blackplanet.com' 20 million African-Americans and many thousands networks more (most figures increasing every second).

'Before speaking first thinking and reading.'
But **WHEN?**

Make your own extra time by adjusting your sleeping pattern as discussed under chapter 14.
"Fast Reading" brings you all knowledge and all the EXTRA time you will need. Today most of us 'slow read' at the speed we speak and that can be enhanced severely, up to 5 times, just imagine, and without losing anything of the meaning or content of the material. Get the first advices from chapter 1 on 'de-stressing', then continue your free search: 'SpeedReadingTrainer.com'

Be a self-confident and convincing speaker:

You will be able to speak load, clear and make your voice indefatigable by a simple exercise.
Kneel in front of a stool put with your hands on your forehead your head on the

cushion. Stretch your knees and legs while inhaling slowly, remain some seconds and come back slowly to your knees while exhaling. Build it up step by step. Later while progressing remove your arms and hands for support. Repeat 3 to 5 times a few times a day, during minimum 21 days and evaluate by singing as loud and long as you want in your car or bathroom. A winner!

At same moment you will build some muscles which are mostly undertrained. Like the 'SCM' (sternocleidomastoid) needed to flex and rotate the head, raising of the sternum and helping with forced inhalation. Or building also some abdominal and leg muscles and. You will find out with the first trial what you can gain.

This exercise will also help with snore-prevention and healing; further details under chapter 14.

So remember say "No, thank you"

        to introvert-ism

        to continued loneliness

But also "YES thank you" to friends, family, ... even enemy

So remember you can add years to your life

        by just listening and observing

        by being socially active

        by helping others

11. Follow their *100+* example

Enough is as good as a feast. ~George Chapman

The value of a long and healthy life is obvious to every reasonable person.

Our limits:
> In the Bible, God declared "My Spirit will not contend with man forever, for he is indeed mortal and their days of life will be 120 years."   ~Genesis 6:3

What factors are most important to achieving maximum lifespan and better health in old age?
Thomas Perls, a geriatrician at the Boston University Medical School, studies centenarians; he has an acronym: AGEING, spelled the British way. "A" is for attitude. Centenarians are optimistic, and they tend to be funny. I think that those personality characteristics translate into being able to manage stress well. They don't internalize stress; they seem to be able to let go. The "G" is for genetics. If people in your family have passed away in their 60s and 70s, alarm bells should be going off: You, more than other people, need to pay attention to prevention and screening. The "E" is for exercise. I say people should exercise five times a week, 30 minutes a day. "I" stands for interest, and that has to do with exercising your brain. "N," nutrition: the goal should be a healthy weight. "G" is for, Get rid of smoking, and get rid of anti-aging quackery. Perls is a very outspoken critic of the anti-aging industry, especially growth hormone, which he thinks is really quite dangerous. Take his Life Expectancy Calculator at 'livingto100.com'.

How has the human life span changed over time?

The same factors that increased lifespan in modern times were also responsible for increasing human life-spans in evolution. Life expectancy doubled from 20 years in our great ape ancestors, to 40 years, which was the general human life expectancy before the modern era.

Caleb Finch, professor of gerontology and biological sciences at the University of Southern California, has spent his scientific career trying to explain why. As a leading researcher on aging and longevity he says: in the last 200 years, one year of extra lifespan has been added for about every four years of historical time. Life expectancy has doubled since the industrial revolution, from about 40 years to near 80 years.

Life expectancy fact: today men in the U.S. can expect to live to age 75.2; women to 81. See also table chapter 25.

'Scientific American' headed in a 10/2008 issue "**Is 100 the new 80?** Healthy aging may be possible with some genetic help"

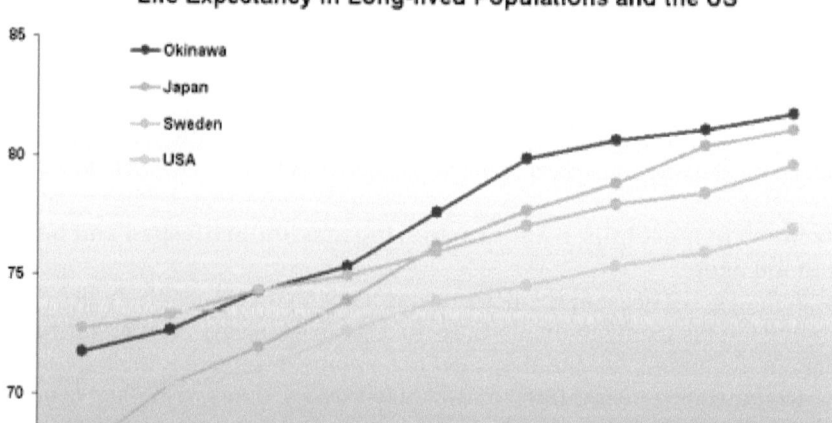

My actual chances to die naturally (not waking up from natural cause) **are 1%!**
From what we die then (in high and middle income countries)?
From chronic diseases. Heart disease, cancer, brain-stroke, Chronic lower respiratory diseases, Accidents (unintentional injuries), Diabetes, Influenza and pneumonia, Alzheimer's disease, Kidney disease and Blood poisoning. They altogether accounted for about 78 percent of all U.S. deaths in 2003. The top two causes, heart disease and cancer, accounted for roughly one-half (50.7 percent) of all deaths in 2003.

What can people do to stay healthy and live longer?

Exercise and maintaining a healthy weight are remarkably preventive for all the diseases of aging. What's good for your heart is good for your brain and is good for preventing cancer. The separate diseases of adult life are much more related to each other and to overall health than we previously recognized. ~Finch; *The Biology of Human Longevity: Inflammation, Nutrition, and Aging in the Evolution of Lifespans -2007*

Hunza centennials until recently were forced to subsist on a Spartan menu of apricots, walnuts, buckwheat cakes and fresh vegetables. They had no other choice.
How they lived? Turn off your electricity, forget heating with coal or oil, no su-

permarket, shopping center, mobile, PC, car, train or plane, hospital, ... survive and imagine.

Are we spoiled or are you spoiling your children?

Minerals in our drinking water: every spring and tap water is different also in relation to minerals. This comparison only shows the differences in total mineral content without detailing the specific minerals in these waters.

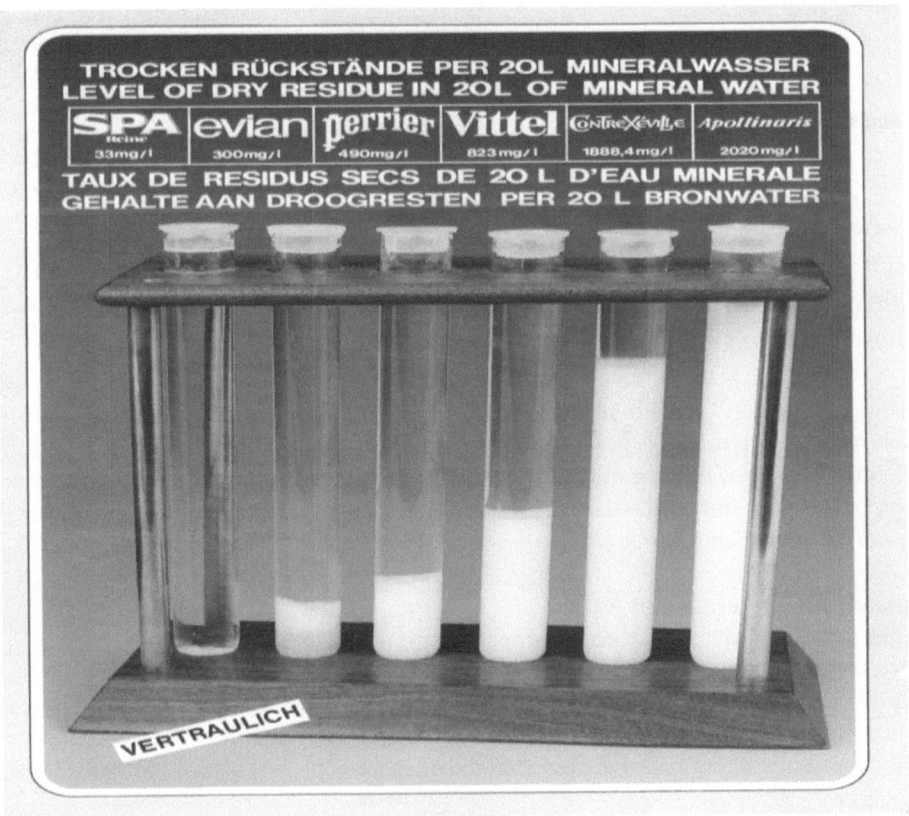

As said earlier water should be **'empty'** so it can clean your body and keep it functioning correctly. That water 'H2O' has **zero calories**, no hazards, only benefits.

"The study of water contains in itself a lesson in humility: all the problems of our knowledge are to be re-examined, reconsidered, according to the realities of the liquid element, essential component of the Earth and Life". ~ Doctor Jeanne Rousseau "Water the Unknown."

Find your origins in the sea!
Rene Quinton (1866-1925), French physiologist and biologist, showed the identity between human blood plasma and seawater, the medium in which life on earth originated and evolved. Quinton extracted seawater from certain areas rich in 'planktonic' life and processed it using his unique protocol. It was referred to as *Plasma de Quinton* or Quinton Marine Plasma. His discovery was put to immediate use in 1905 as the pandemics of cholera, tuberculosis, typhoid, syphilis and smallpox descended upon Europe. Through government cooperation, sixty-nine Marine Dispensaries were established throughout Europe, as well as in Cairo and Algiers, to treat the diseased population. Hundreds of thousands of lives were saved using this natural substance until the outbreak of WWI. Quinton Marine Plasma was then successfully used as a blood plasma replacement in both World Wars.

The human body is 65-70% water in the form of vital blood plasma, lymph, extracellular and interstitial fluids, which have essentially the same composition and infinitesimal structure as seawater. Often referred to as the human "terrain", it is believed that the health and balance of these fluids can be restored and maintained by the proper application of Quinton Marine Plasma.

Original Quinton™ marine plasma is available as hypertonic or isotonic nutrient-rich marine matrix that is harvested from the depths of an oceanic plankton bloom. It has proven to be an effective way to restore cellular homeostasis, repolarization and mineral balance. For details: 'originalquinton.com', or for Europe 'quinton.es' and 'quinton.fr'.

Absorbable **Minerals and Aging:**
Aging studies show a close tie to mineral content and use in the body. A particularly interesting study explored the possible reasons why several societies around the world had healthy life spans exceeding those of industrialized societies. The purpose of studying these societies was to consider any possible link between these societies' aging and their foods and drinks.

Among the societies studied were the Hunzas of Northern Pakistan, the Vilcabamba tribe from Ecuador and a community living on the island of Okinawa in Japan. The Hunzas, the study noted, routinely had several citizens reaching the age of +100!

Dr Coanda discovered that the secret of longevity of **the Hunzas** was due to the special physical properties of their water. The people who live in these areas also claim that water is the secret of their long, healthy lives. He found that this 'Hunza-type' water was significantly different from water found anywhere else.

Dr. Coanda told Dr Patrick Flanagan: "Discover the secret of Hunza -type water and you can extend life indefinitely." Dr Flanagan discovered that Hunza water is in many ways just like distilled water. It does not contain the mineral salts found in some mountain springs or in well water. It is devoid of mineral salts. It would also have a different spin (left turning) than most other waters.

Hunza water contains trace minerals (mainly silica and silver) in a special colloidal form. Colloidal minerals are minerals that are insoluble in water. Colloidal minerals are not ionized into anions and cations like mineral salts. Although colloidal minerals are very common types of minerals, the colloids in Hunza water are different from ordinary colloids. Colloidal minerals are so tiny that they cannot be seen except with the most powerful microscopes. Instead of being ionized, they are suspended in water by a phenomenon known as "zeta potential". For so far the Doctors Coanda and Flanagan.

We measured ourselves samples of many spring, tap, well and bottled waters so also the Hunza water and found it indeed having a milky appearance due to the colloids and the total mineral content was 90 ppm (mg/l). Glacier water and mountain spring water at the source all have a very high content of free electrons, expressed through their negative ORP or low rH_2, thus are '**reduced**' . They flow within granite rock and contain loads of Silicium, but at the same moment have a very low total mineral content (always below 100 ppm).

The Vilcabamba tribe boasts 16 of the 800 people over the age of 100 years! The tribe's average cholesterol count is 80 points lower than the US average and heart disease, cancer and diabetes are virtually unknown.

When the researchers looked at the mineral content in the bodies of all participants, they noted an extremely rich source of calcium, magnesium and other significant trace minerals. With the exception of the group of **Okinawan** Japanese, these communities are from mountainous regions. The study noted that the mineral-rich water used for irrigation and drinking, deriving from glaciers, could be the bond that liked the aging phenomenon, but this did not account for the group from Okinawa.

In studying the water source, the minerals from the glaciers were laden with these life-sustaining minerals. This led to the question of the mineral source in the Japanese. The researchers discovered that the group of Okinawan's regularly fertilized their soil with pulverized mineral-rich coral reefs.

The researchers found the common denominator - the high mineral content of all the study cultures must account for their incredible longevity. Later studies confirmed these results and signify the link between minerals and aging.

Since most of us are not able to live in areas enriched with glacier-fed water or reef-fertilized soils, we must look for alternatives to provide the body with highly absorbable minerals.

Dr. Flanagan patented his findings within his 'Crystal energy', for more details: 'wetterwater.net'.

Let it be clear that for me (*) in any 'centenarian-' or 'Blue Zone' it is not about the drinking water only, be it even and of course pure, dynamic, untreated, with low mineral content and balanced.
These waters were indeed un-comparable with any known tap- or bottled water from our 'civilized' world.
(*)*tropical agriculture engineer, able to observe in the 70-ies for years mountain Berber tribes in Morocco, formerly and first European member of the US Water Quality Association being Certified Water Specialist level V, trained BEV-specialist.*

BUT it is, and honestly more and more 'was', also and simultaneously about:

- **ZERO** vaccins, pasteurization, preservatives, additives, refined sugar, refined flour, chemicals, pesticides, hormones, electricity, war, crime, toothpaste, smoothies, retirement, …

- **Little** meat or fish (grilled or raw), butter or grease, alcohol, calories, time and distance between field harvesting and consumption, emotional stress, disputes, the right genes (*)

- **Maximum** survival (of the fittest), fermented, raw, ripe seasonal fruit, vegetables and nuts, whole grain, pure air and full breathing, sunshine, moderation, physical effort (walking long distances, field and housework), social contact, respect of elderly and nature, balance with cosmos, simple and pure thinking (mind controls body),optimism and spring fasting.

And **optimal energy vibrations** in water, food, air, light and people's minds.

(*)**Genes are segments of DNA.** Genes are found in chromosomes and they control growth and help you stay healthy. Tests can give indications on your metabolism of lipids, obesity, inflammation and anti-oxidant activity. **Nutrigenetics** studies the relationship between genes and diet, with the goal to optimize health through the personalization of our diet. Get the why and how on gene testing: 'aimo.it'.

Further we should know about ongoing longevity myths:

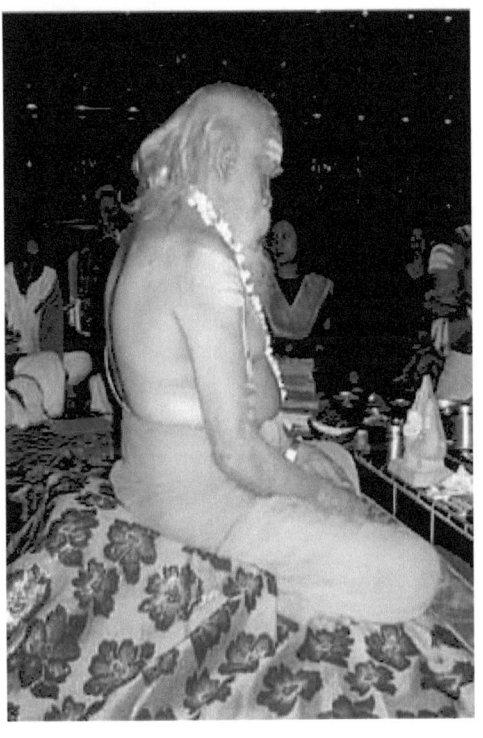

- Only approximately fifty people in human history have been documented as reaching the age of 114.
- Only about twenty of those people who reached 114 have reached the age of 115.
- Of the eight people regarded by the Guinness Book or significant scholars to have reached 116, three are subject to substantial doubt.
- Jeanne Calment is the only person absolutely undisputed to have lived to or over 120.
- Recently (07/2010) Sri Swami Buaji Maharaj (see his picture on the left), passed away at 120+ years of age (born 1889) he kept all along a sharp mind and body supple and full of life.

"Begin the day with love, spend the day with love, fill the day with love, end the day with love. That is the way to God." ~ Maha YogiRaj Sri Swami Buaji

What the centenarian communities of the Vilcabamba valley in Equador, Azerbeidjan, Kreta, Sardinia, Morocco Atlas ,... have in common is also a lot of sunshine, nice Springs and long warm Summers, crisp air and breathtaking blue skies, sunsets and sun-takes, nature noises or silence and a glittering Milky Way galaxy and universe at night. In other words: an almost romantic, peaceful, mystic and low-stress environment. Further they never retired and kept on fighting the elements to survive.

True, modern science, food-industry, medicine and pharma-chemicals keep more of us longer on our feet than ever before, but at what a cost as well financially as environmentally. Also remains the client, consumer or patient confused or uninformed about the global outcome for his healthy aging.

Okinawa: researchers found their subjects ate about 20% fewer calories than the Japanese average; which in turn is about 20% lower than the average in the U.S. The Okinawan elders who were part of Suzuki's study got most of their protein from fish, which provides another so-called good fat: omega-3. This oil is particularly prevalent in fish such as salmon, tuna and mackerel, whose established heart-protecting properties are considered by researchers to be an important reason that Japan's incidence of heart disease is one-third that of the U.S.'s. Okinawans have about one-fifth as many heart attacks as North Americans, Suzuki says, and when they do, they are twice as likely to survive. "Okinawa's national dish is a stir-fry called *chample*," says Suzuki. "The exact recipe varies from house to house but the basic ingredients are always there: tofu, soya beans and *goya* [a local variety of bitter gourd]. Those three are all very high in flavonoids as well as other compounds like isoflavones, saponins and vitamins B and C that provide protection against free radicals."Further did the researchers conclude: "we believe the Okinawans have both genetic and non-genetic longevity advantages -- the best combination. In fact, we have written extensively that the Okinawan traditional way of life -- the dietary habits, the physical activity, the psychological and social aspects, all play an important role in Okinawan longevity". ~ 'okicent.org'

These Japanese, who consume large amounts of 'fermented' soy foods like natto and miso along with green tea, ginger and ocean herbs, have the longest lifespan of any people in the world.

Dr. Weston A. Price found among his studies of 14 tribal diets that they provided almost complete immunity to tooth decay and resistance to disease. These diets contained no refined or devitalized foods. Contact with civilization, followed by adoption of the "displacing foods of modern commerce," was disastrous for all groups studied. 'ppnf.org'

Scientists generally agree that less than 25 percent of how long we live is dictated by **genetics** -- how long our parents and grandparents lived. The other 75 percent or so is determined by our lifestyle -- our habits day-in and day-out.

You want to know how long the Social Security statistics you still grants? Check your actual age on the list and find out: 'ssa.gov'

Have a look (page 143) at the US Census Bureau's 'Population Pyramid' comparison for the years 2000, 2025 and 2050. Look how the 85+ figures quadruple, not to say are going through the pyramids roof (as extension till +110 years will be needed)! Or look at the dynamic comparison from 1955 till 2050 and watch the real slender pyramid grow out of proportion into a massive block, more and more dominated by the 3rd and 4th generations:
'census.gov/cgi-bin/ipc/idbpyrs.pl?cty=US&out=d&ymax=250&submit=Envoyer' .

My founding example: Prof. **Paul Bouts**, Belgian phrenologist and pedagogue. Internationally known for his characterological analysis and theories, which he coined **Psychognomy**. He experienced serious health problems, due to overburdening in his 50-ies. He then studied a healthy lifestyle, which he described in his work *Modern Hygiene of Intellectuals*. He underlined the importance of wholesome, healthy food and of the maintenance of respiratory capacity through exercise. Already in the 1960-ties he opened a since then renowned reform shop called 'Sol&Vita'. The adoption of this healthy lifestyle allowed him to regain **full strength** and to lead a **productive life** beyond age 99 when he passed away with a smile on his face. **Thank you 'professor'** for showing us that change, moderation, balanced food intake, exercise, reflection and helping others do make the difference in life.

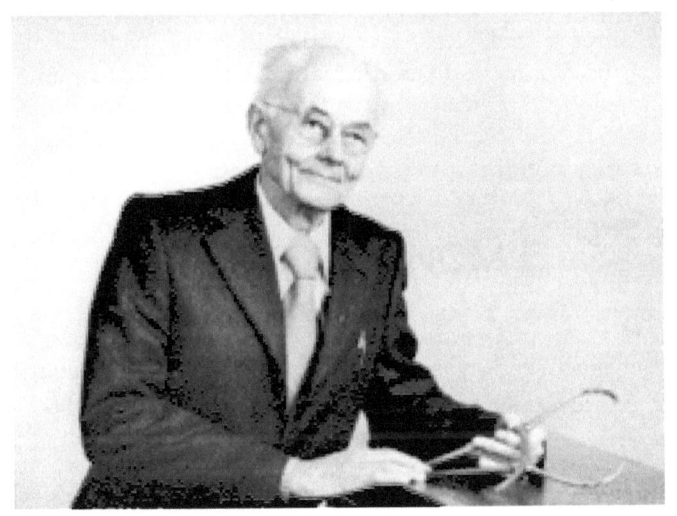

I also want to honor a great nonagerian **Dr. Jeanne Rousseau**, born 02-01 1915, pioneer in the 1950-ies, with Professor Louis Claude Vincent on the Bio-electronic science, and today honorable president of the Bio-Electronic society and honorable member of the Biophysical Comity of **the World Academy of Bio-Medical Technology**/Unesco. All her life she was a model of intellectual probity, moral rigor and will. She stayed magnificently active till 2007 and not capitulating till this very day. As a researcher she wrote numerous articles such as on 'Water, the unknown', 'Cosmic resonances' and 'Hydrospire, the vitalizing bath'. Some of her quotations: "Water, air, land, fire, blood, sap of the plants they are all structured elements to the image of the universe. This structure, which channels the mysterious vital force, is probably no other than the 'ether', unknown to date".

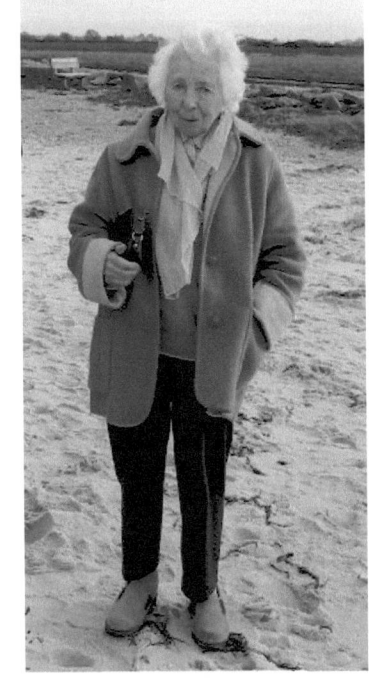

"The Fountain of Youth, the formerly myth, will she be the scientific reality of tomorrow? Will we see re-blossom the old hope, deeply rooted in the heart of man: that of being able to live its entire life, while ignoring, like the Hunzas, the debilitating influence of old age, of the pathological degeneration and of the pain?" Dr. Jeanne Rousseau, written 09/67. **Thank you Doctor Jeanne**, for showing us your beautiful and ongoing biography and remembering us that: **"When a scientific theory does not correspond to reality, the theory must be considered false and rejected, while the reality remains and is to be imposed"**.

Find your star, your example: 'genarians.com' or follow the stories of the World's **'Blue Zones'** where people always get older than average 'bluezones.com'.

What they say:
"The secret to long life is being active, (if) you keep your mind busy and keep your body busy, you're going to be around a long time." Walter Breuning born 09- 1896.

"Children and adults should eat fruit instead of drinking fruit juices and drink only water." On her 100th birthday in 1998, she refused cake as there was too much sugar in it. Leila Denmark born 02-1898.

"Love everybody, treat everybody right, never drink or smoke." Maggie Renfro born 11-1895

"When you use your brains, they just get sharper. Everything is recorded up there; you don't have to make it up." Frederica Sagor Maas born born 07-1900

My LONGEVITY I attribute to, number one, EXCESSIVE EXERCISE! On business trips to Los Angeles, I would carry my own bags -- from the airport to downtown, walking all 18 miles (30 kilometer!). At 82, he ran the London Marathon -- and finished in a little more than six hours. Albert Gordon born 07-1901

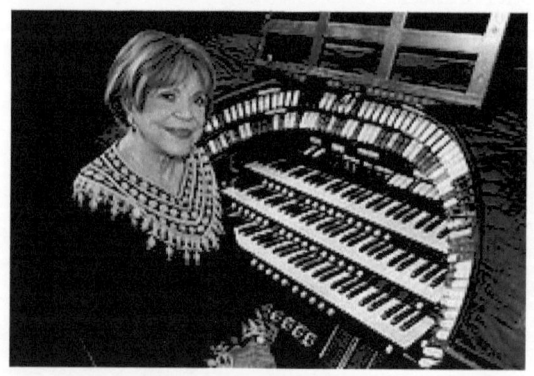

Rosa Rio born 06-1902 look and listen for yourself

'youtube.com/ watch?v=kA6uNNmCYe8'

She shows with conviction that there is **quality of live** beyond 100!

Aged 112, actual oldest man in India. Pandit Sudhakar Chaturvedi of Bangalore (born there in 1897) says the secret of his long life is laughing, loving, strict vegetarian diet, vitamin tablets and a passion for the Vedas. "If one follows the Vedas and **keep one's body, soul and speech pure**, a healthy long life is in store for him," he says. This sprightly centenarian gives lectures, writes articles, is a consultant and walks around comfortably with a walking stick. He works for eight hours every day. He gets up at 3.30 am and starts reading the Upanishads and darshans. Two hours are kept aside for meditation. He reads newspapers and magazines in English, Hindi and Kannada and discusses the reports with visitors. "I want to be happy and **make others happy** - that's my whole aim of living now," said Chaturvedi.

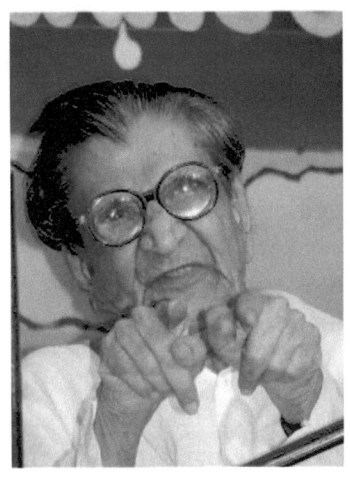

Keizo Miura *(1904-2006)*, shown here doing part of his **daily exercise routine**. Every morning he moves his neck left and right about **100 times**, opens his mouth wide and **sticks out his tongue** to train his face and mouth muscles. He says this is to prevent bagginess around the mouth, which is prevalent among elderly people. He also does squats and other exercises to strengthen his body, and **walks about 3-4 kilometers each day**. He was notable for his fitness and outdoor-sport undertakings **at advanced age**; he was the oldest person to climb the Kilimanjaro, at age 77 and descended a Mont Blanc glacier of the age 99 together with his oldest son and grandson. On February 15, 2004, Keizo celebrated his centennial birthday with a ski descent together with more than 170 friends and family members, including four generations of his family, at Snowbird ski resort in Salt

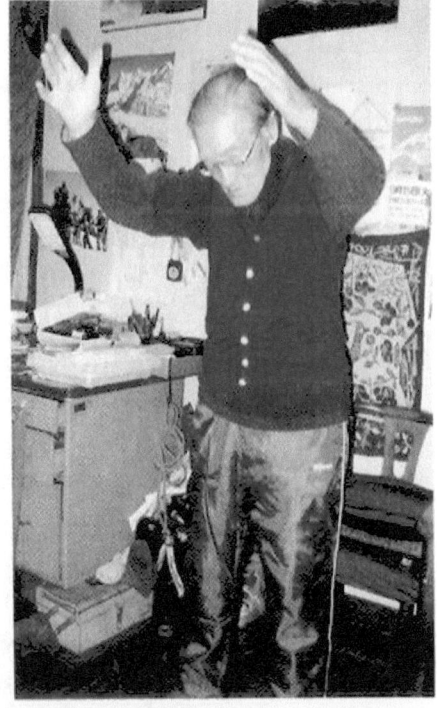

Lake City. His **main diet** consisted of unpolished rice mixed with whole rice, which becomes sweet if it is **chewed well**. He also ate **fish**, preparing it in a pressure cooker to make the bony parts soft and edible. To help his body absorb the calcium from the bones, he said he ate wood ear mushrooms, which are rich in **vitamin D**. Other items on Miura's menu included hijiki, a type of edible **seaweed**, and **fermented** soybeans. He says he tries to eat **several kinds** of foods in each meal. After breakfast and dinner he has a nutritional drink containing sesame **seeds**, soybean flour, **yogurt** and milk. What a summary! What an example! **Thank You Keizo.**

Well they all were or still are dynamic, slim and in balance during their entire or second half of their life! Agree?

The 'Western' centenarians have worked at heavy physical labor their entire lives and most still do. They all have a strong and supportive social structure. All remain active in their community, they are surrounded by people who care about them and that they care about.
The centenarians tend to have a lower level of stress in their lives and the hard work tends to help them burn off what stress they have. While they do eat meat, it is not a daily component of their diets.

From present data, the number of worldwide Centenarians is around 450,000. By 2050, "the number of US centenarians alone is expected to reach 834,000 and maybe even 1 million," said Dr. Robert Butler, President of the International Longevity Center in New York City.

Still don't know where and how long to go, then remember where you come from and feel assured you will not be alone then.

What we can deduct as 'MUST-DO' from the centenarian* history/experience:

1) Deep breath exercises with integration in your daily routine and the use of an in-house air-purifier/-ionizer or sufficient oxygenating plants compensates for the pure mountain air Hunza, Vilcabamba, Azerbeidjani, Atlas-Berber and most past centenarians were inhaling their entire life
2) Eating with <u>moderation</u> and in peace with time and environment, no fried food but seasonal veggies, including onion and garlic, seasonal fruits and nuts and rarely meat to imitate our high valley examples
3) Walk daily in nature under any condition be it snow, rain , wind or sun as they did

4) Work-out/Exercise +4x/week for minimum 30' to imitate part of the intensive physical labor they did their entire life (no retirement)
5) Drink up to 0.5gln/2lt of pure (R.O.) water/day as such or partly as herbal tea or extra energized to copy their source of vital, living, low mineral glacier water
6) Kefir, yoghourt and other fermented products (like the Lesik® 'ferments of life') which they used daily
7) Respect and communicate with family, neighbors, ... and network to follow their healthy intense socializing habits
8) No alcohol or moderately and rarely during special meetings
9) Organic forest fruits, bitter almonds, seeds of apricot (B17), supplements to get your daily anti-oxidants intake
10) See how you can assimilate the fact that they had untreated drinking water and limited amount of natural grown foods much less comfort and income but more air, space, time, contact with the elements and with their fellow tribe people

*which might have been nonagenarians, but still hats off considering their difficult living conditions.

So remember say "No, thank you"
to pessimism
to most out of the 'zero'-list

So remember you can add years to your life
by practicing the above 'Must-do"

12. Enjoy a healthy partner-, sex- and family live

A heart that loves is always young.   *Greek Proverb*

Love yourself first! Impossible to find the one you are made for and to make that someone happy if you are not in balance yourself.
Accept yourself first as you are then build your self-esteem. Think what makes you unique. Learn from your shortcomings and build on your strengths. Think positive about yourself.

No clue?

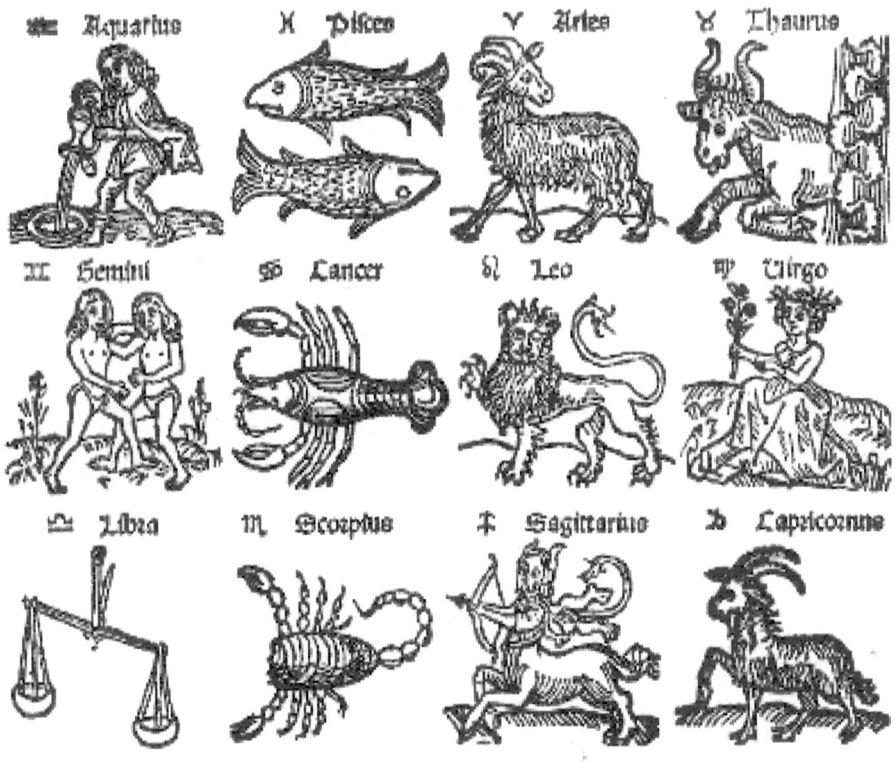

Find and read a good book on your 'horoscope' sign or have a 'Numerology' reading. Yes it is all about **cosmic energy** and the exact minute, hour, day, month and year you were born. You can get started here: astrology-online.com . It is not about believe it is about your place in the universe.

The three main traditions of astrology, the Western, Indian and Chinese, share the same fundamental idea of a twelve sign zodiac with the signs divided into four basic types.
It is not about promises it is about your 'specific' figures.

Western Sign Element	Indian Sign Element	Chinese Sign Trine
Aries Fire	**Mesha** Tejas (fire)	**Dragon** (5) 1st
Taurus Earth	**Vrishabha** Prithivi (earth)	**Snake** (6) 2nd
GeminiAir	**Mithuna**Vayu (air)	**Horse** (7)3rd
CancerWater	**Karka**Jala (water)	**Sheep** (8)4th
LeoFire	**Simha**Tejas (fire)	**Monkey** (9)1st
VirgoEarth	**Kanya**Prithivi (earth)	**Rooster** (10)2nd
LibraAir	**Tula**Vayu (air)	**Dog** (11)3rd
ScorpioWater	**Vrishchika**Jala (water)	**Pig** (12)4th
SagittariusFire	**Dhanus**Tejas (fire)	**Rat** (1)1st
CapricornEarth	**Makara**Prithivi (earth)	**Ox** (2)2nd
AquariusAir	**Kumbha**Vayu (air)	**Tiger** (3)3rd
PiscesWater	**Meena**Jala (water)	**Rabbit** (4)4th

It is more than just prediction. Accurately calculated calendars exist since millennia. Hindu's Purana predicted 4 different cycles which could be **the Galactic Cycle**, Kali being the last one with a time span of 4,32,000 years. The Maya's had their solar and other calendars. According to Aztec cosmology, the universe is in a very delicate equilibrium.

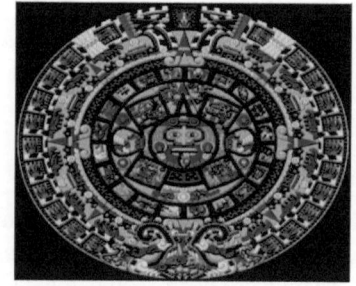

Find the right partner(s). Know or learn about your preferences. **Monogamy** can work out fantastical, but it is since **recent it became dominant** to serve mainly traditional, historical, religious, social and economical purposes in our Western society, just like polygamy was since ever and still is in different cultures. Abraham was in digamy (remarried), which is not bigamy. Polygyny (one man has more than one wife) is dominant but polyandry (one woman having more than one man) and group marriage remains. A survey of **traditional societies** in the world shows that 83.39% of them practice **polygyny**, 16.14% practice monogamy, and .47% practice polyandry. **Polyandry** has been or still is practiced in India, Tibet, Nepal, Bhutan, Sri Lanka, parts of the Arctic, areas of Mongolia and in some African and American indigenous groups. It is also thought to have been consumed in some Polynesian communities. It was mostly 'outlawed', but is still socially accepted.

What to look for in a partner: don't stop with the look and cuteness, use your instinct. Honesty from both sides will save time and energy. Readiness to listen to each other, to show mutual respect and to have an open friendly communication. Joyfulness. Flexibility. Truthfulness. Optimistic. Forgiving. Fullness. Add your other preferences, but find out first if you demonstrate those qualities yourself. The more you learned about yourself the easier for you to understand what the other is looking for. Be open minded and you will see the abundance in the other. They will bring you the missing pieces in your puzzle of life. The search is in you. Focus and you will attract. Again all knowledge and answers are already within you, just clear your mind and deep breathe. It is all about energy and vibrations, stay tuned and in balance.

Where to find a partner: they can and will come out of the blue which is perfect and trilling.
The "Law of Attraction" (*) explains that everything is interconnected. It's all about you and you can have everything your heart desires. As said search inside yourself, think your dream and go on. Otherwise as usual at work, college, university, friends, family, matchmaking, church, sports, hobbies, parties, clubs, going for a drink, internet, chat, … According to industry surveys, more than 22million people visited dating websites in 2007. Visitors are on average 55% male and thus 45% female. Why not: 'match.com', 'datingdirect.com', 'singlesnet.com', 'plentyoffish.com', 'personals.yahoo.com', 'americansingles.com', 'eharmony.com', 'seniorfriendfinder.com', 'asianfriendsearch.com', 'indianfriendsearch.com' and a 1000 more.
(*) recently over-Buzzed as practiced since eternity, but if not yet informed and motivated, start reading "The Secret"~Rhonda Byrne, Atria Books 2006 or watch 'thesecret.tv'.

Look your be-loved people in the eyes and repeat, also after many years, the words used at your first important meeting or wedding. Not always easy as it stays an experiment partnering or 'marriage'.
Give them time for self-development, air to breathe, ...be empathic.

Keep perspective. Nobody is supposed to be perfect.

> Be flexible
> > Accept some dogma and relativize others
> > Do not stop learning from each other
> Stay young at heart

Cushion fight instead of word- or psycho fighting. By the way you burn 26 calories in a one-minute kiss.

Sex means not 'as usual' or uni-directed (penis/him first)

> Get informed about the many positions and plays and then forget about it (Chinese, Indian/Kama Sutra,... old knowledge by text and/or drawings) as it is more about feeling, acting, practicing and repeating then reading or talking about it. Many African tribes had and still have initiation rites where elderly family members (aunts/uncles) teach their off-spring hands on how to sexually act.

So what if the grass is greener ... after some time ...resource yourself and stay on the hill. Give and take freedom when needed, but in consent.

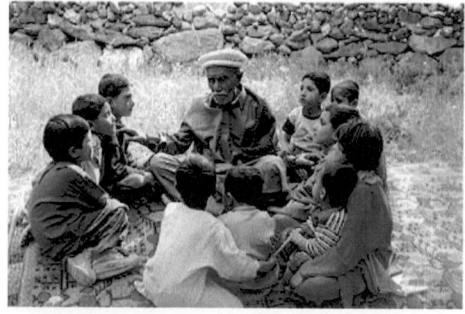

Family means not children first. Grandparents, parents, children, grandchildren have all a place and roll in a balanced life pattern. Children should be taken care of but not be spoiled in a world which is more 'flat' and competitive than ever.

Family and friends: A good friend can help keep the doctor away. Harvard researchers investigated the effect of social ties, death and heart disease. Socially isolated men were 53% more likely to die from a heart-related cause than those who reported the highest number of social ties. Overall, married men reportedly had a lower risk of death from any cause and a greater than twofold reduced risk of death from accidents and suicides than their unmarried peers. Social isolation is a 'risk factor' for ill health.

But When? Reduce the amount of money you have to earn (*), you'll have a lot more freedom to do the things you love, and more freedom to spend time with the people you love.
(*) or find ways to be more productive in less working hours, read also chapter 2.
If your life is always hectic, if you don't have friends, if you're doing work you don't really like, then **change**.

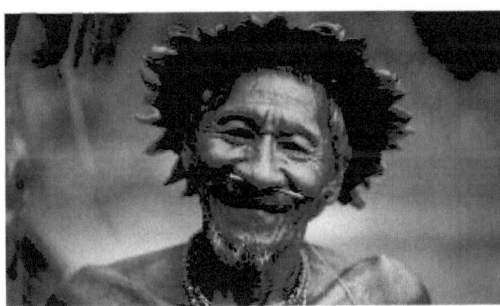

Tribal societies, as those where the "centenarians" live(d), were known to behave very socially ....read also chapter 10, get informed and active : sur'vival-international.org'

Getting in touch is a start, but meeting the 'other' is the real goal. It is you and only you who holds the 'connection' key. Your traditional social network size is limited to about 150 persons. Using your PC you can crank up your communication level easy to an average of 1900 email-contacts.

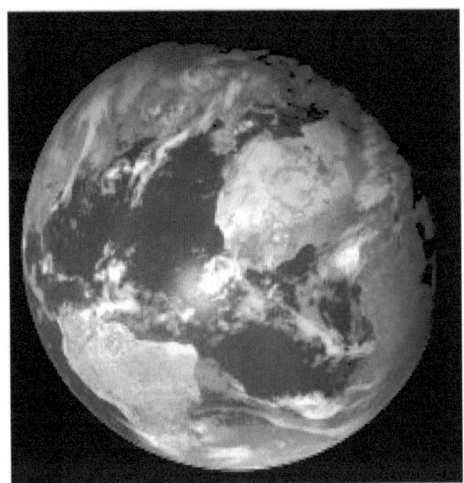

The   is yours.

Some figures about **modern networking** (needing continuous updating as growing too fast): there are

701 million mailboxes worldwide

232 million emails send, thus also received a day

72% of them are spam

37% of US citizens get and read news/information on-line

550 years after Gutenberg started printing it is all getting paperless: ticketing, classroom, boarding, immigration, news, punching, office, reading (*), agenda, billing, paying, be paid, ... (**)

(*) number of FREE-Ebook downloads at www.gutenberg.org : a day in the spring 2009: 100191, last 7 days 639 192 last 30 days 2 648 477!

This just as a first motivational prove and to compensate you for your investment in this book; the latter in case you would not find any other interesting topic/subject/advice in mine; then search another book for free among the 27.000 available and growing in over 40 languages of your choice (***). RELAX!

(**) have your spam filter installed and your back-ups made

(***) give them a hand and proof-read a page a day ; oxygenates your brain and makes you feel good on top

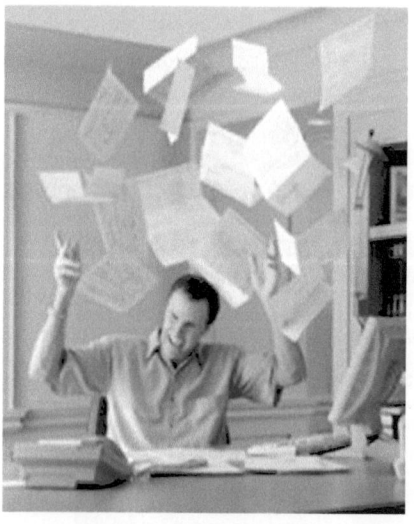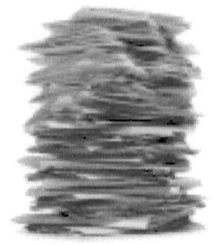

Think about the environment before printing this e-mail 🌐

Log-in to our newsletter/ blog and find continuous updates   'enjoyvity.com'

Your Natural and Free Viagra!

Increase you marital or partner joy. Many advices given in the **"EnjoyVity"** book as on healthy eating, drinking and thinking can help you enjoy a better sex life because it will increase your blood flow, general health and your self-image. Here some extra and specific exercises to keep and build or rebuild tonus within and among your sex organs at any age. Here also 'rest brings rust' and it is never too late to start!

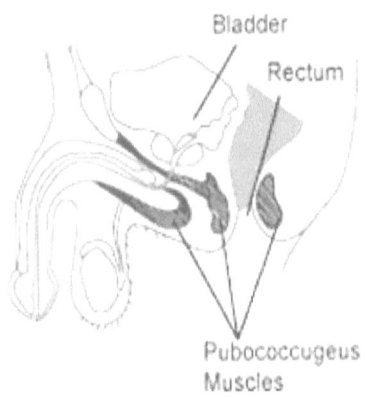

He: 'squeeze and relax' your anus muscles (the old Chinese 'pubis squeeze'). Men with a strong PC muscle can enjoy more sensation in their genital area, better ejaculation control, stronger orgasms and even **better prostate health**. Build your perineum muscles, as if you want to hold or interrupt urinating or stools. You feel your anus closing and your sexual organs moving slightly. Alternate, squeezing and relaxing, every some seconds. Build it up step by step towards a tempo of 3 seconds 50x and 6x/day. For more details, also on the slow squeeze where you combine muscle movements with deep diaphragm breathing, read 'the yin-yang butterfly' ~ Valentin Chu, Putnam's NY

She: the Kegel exercises. Women with a strong PC (PuboCoccugeus) muscle, which make up the pelvic floor, have many benefits, including toning the vagina after giving birth, controlling your bladder and making it easier for you to have orgasms. Here's how: when you're peeing, clench your muscles to stop the flow of urine for about four seconds. Then release those same muscles to let the urine flow again. These are your pelvic floor muscles; another technique to find them: insert a finger inside your vagina and try to squeeze the surrounding muscles. You

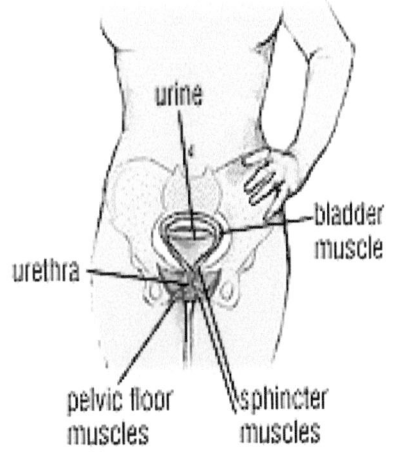

should be able to feel your vagina tighten and your pelvic floor move upward. These are the muscles you'll be exercising when you do 'Kegel's'. Be careful not to flex the muscles in your abdomen, thighs or buttocks. About five to ten times a day, repeat the 'Kegel's' ten times per session. Can be done at any moment in the car, office, TV-watching, …; try for 2 months and evaluate with your partner. More to learn: 'kegel-exercises.com'

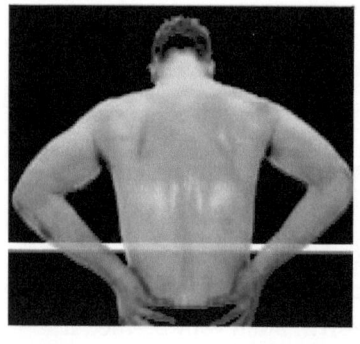

He&she: Build also your abdomen, belly and back muscles to improve your look and avoid back pain. Note that **80% of people** suffer from back pain at some point in their lives. Find soft exercises to restore strength for lower back and to tone other muscles and maintain strong bones at 'orthoinfo.aaos.org', also for elderly and about your back and strengthening the muscles that support the spine 'bigbackpain.com'.

Combination with 'Kuhne' cold packaging (chapter 8), weight control, sporty-exercises and some deep stomach breaths will do the unexpected at the needed moments.

So remember say "No, thank you"
        to spoiling children

        to back pain

So remember you can add years to your life
        by building your PC's

        by loving yourself

13. Auto diagnose and Self-treat

**Enjoy convalescence. It is the part that makes the illness worthwhile.
~George Bernard Shaw**

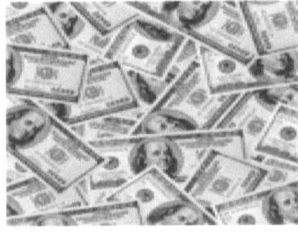

Save some money on your health budget: Americans annually spend $5,267 per capita on health care, while the industrialized world's median is $2,193. Prevention is key.

According to Ayurveda (science of life), excessive use, inadequate use and improper use of food (intakes), physical activities, mental activities or behavior are the causes of all diseases. Learn about the balanced world of 'the Knowledge of Life' which is the Ayurveda since over 5000 years, at 'indiashopping.net'

We can learn about, and get relief from many acute or chronic problems while practicing tongue diagnosis, auriculo-therapy (ear) or iridology (eye) and reflex zone therapy (foot). A normal tongue is reddish, supple and clear without a coating. Get an intro from the world's specialist 'giovanni-maciocia.com'.

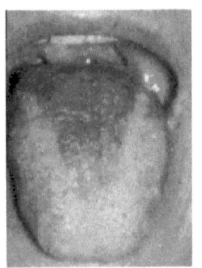

Is it all Chinese?

Acupressure, shiatsu or reflexology: or 'digitopuncture' stimulation of the points of acupuncture with the fingers, finds its origins in the Indian Ayurveda and later the Chinese extended it further. Physical pressure is applied to known acupuncture points by the hand. Specific acupressure points have particular organs associated with them. If somebody has a problem of constipation, there will be a particular type of pain on pressing the associated acupressure points. Frequently press these points regularly and the pain goes away along with the disease. There is no pain at these points in healthy individuals.

Foot: every organ in our thorax can be traced and stimulated at the palm of our feet

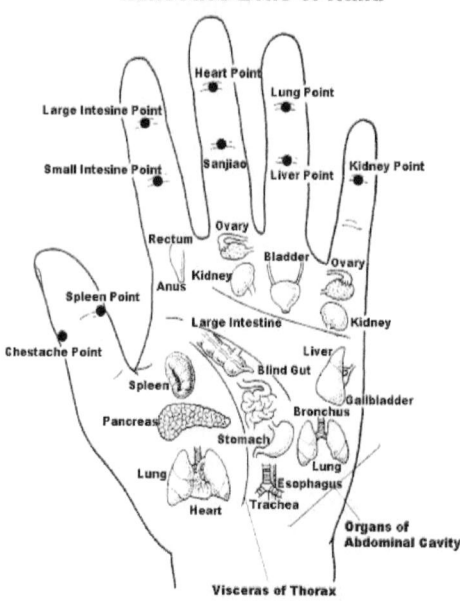

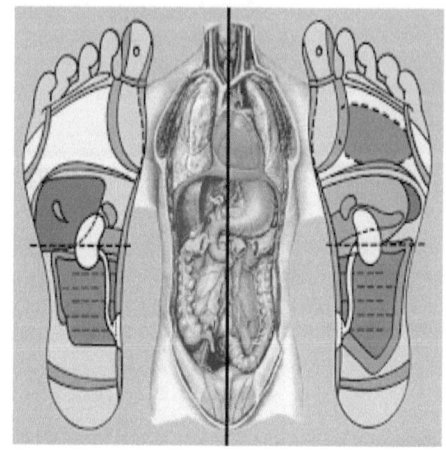

Thus apply pressure there on your feet where you may have pain or have health problems in your body and find instant relief.

Hand: massage of your hand-palm stimulates acu-points on the hand, which will restore the **flow of energy** and thus facilitates body circulation, promotes metabolism and improves immunity function (also great when overusing PC-keyboard and mouse).

Dr. Reinhold Voll, a German physician stated: "pain is the tissue's cry for energy". If there is pain, there is certainly not enough energy.

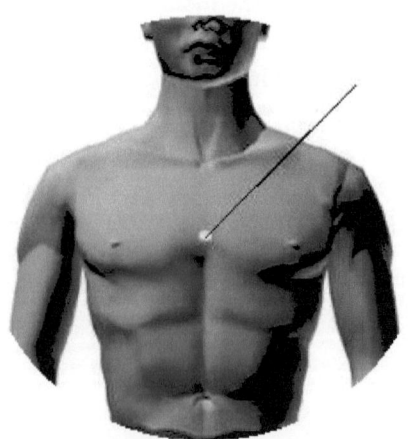

Stress: Try the gentle placement with light pressure of your fingertips on the area of the 'Sea of Tranquility' point (SOT-point, see yellow dot) along with a few slow gentle stomach breaths in and out, and see if this brings you into a calmer state. If it does, you can use this technique to help you get to **sleep** at night, to **reduce stress** while at work, in the daily traffic jam and at any time when you need a gentle reminder to restore calm.

We know there are few physiological functions unaffected by our mental-emotional state. Double-check and practice 'EFT', details in chapter 9.

Applied kinesiology: is a form of diagnosis using muscle testing as a primary feedback mechanism to examine how a person's body is functioning. Its also a therapy wherein the practitioner applies light finger-tip massage to pressure points on the body or head in order to stimulate or relax key muscles. In some cases, the examiner may test for environmental or food sensitivities by using a previously strong muscle to find what weakens it. Learn more about the 'wholistic health model': 'synergistickinesiology.com' and at 'relfe.com'.

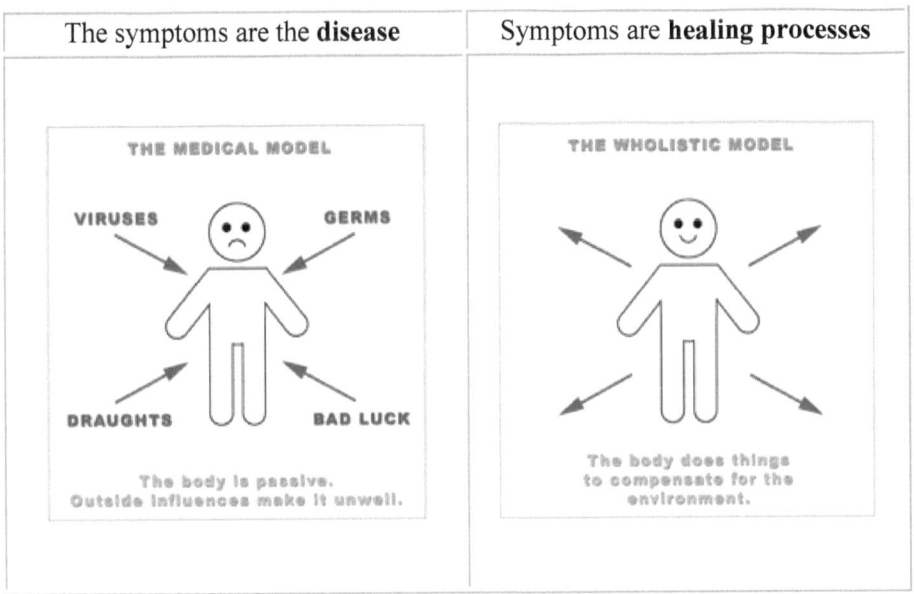

Read also on Educational-Kinesiology for relieving learning disorders and behaviors. See chapter 9.

Don't know yet? Find out if **Your Symptoms** are due to a **Hormonal Imbalance**. Women can have an excess or deficiency in progesterone or estrogen or other imbalances, but also men can have testosterone deficiencies or estrogen excesses. Saliva testing is a simple, accurate way to determine your "free" or bio-available hormone levels, read more: 'johnleemd.com'.

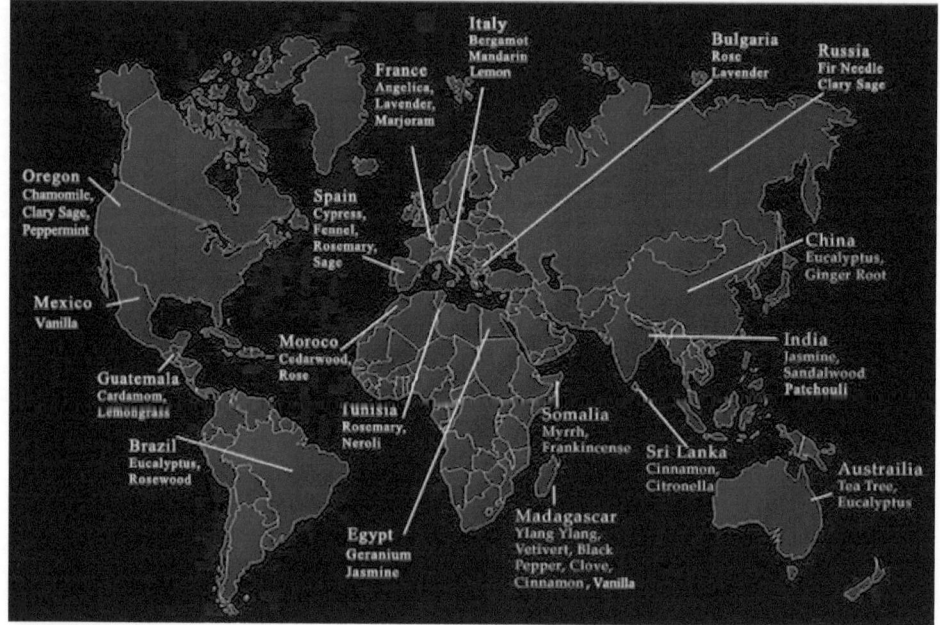

Aroma-therapy: The use of volatile plant oils, including essential oils, distilled from plants that come from every continent on the globe, for psychological and physical well-being. Each plant shares a vibrant aromatic energy. The oils are mainly used in diffusers to create a room mist, or in bath and shower products, but can also be scented. Try a drop in your hand palm, rub and inhale with a deep breath. There are oils to inspire, balance, soothe, meditate, purify, relax, clarify, ... more 'aromatherapy.com'.

Homeopathics: are safe, effective, holistic and natural remedies. The remedies are taken in an extremely diluted form as one part of the remedy for 1 trillion parts of water and are based on the principle 'like cures like'. Homeopathy is the second most widely used system of medicine in the world. Try the '**online remedy finder**' at 'abchomeopathy.com'.

Your smile and you: your smile expresses who you are and how you feel. Don't hide your happiness. We can all agree that a whiter, brighter smile can make you look younger, healthier, more inviting, and more confident. DIY or get a good dentist.

The 'Kegel's' don't forget; reread under chapter 12 and practice daily.

Move, exercise, practice yoga,...

Breath well
Breathing is the main connection between the mind and body. You need to take time to slow down your breathing and observe it: breathe in and breathe out. By coming to your breath, you can calm your emotions and stay in the present moment. Some yogis, many of whom live well beyond age 100, have slowed their breathing to four or five breaths a minute, and a recent study by the Santa Fe Institute, an independent research and education center, connects the slower pulse rates of the world's larger mammals to their expanded life-spans. Most of us breathe (through our mouth mainly) using our upper chest and this is not right. Breathing correctly shall not only help the body take in more oxygen, it will also help you burn more calories, speed up your metabolism, which in turn, helps you burn more fats.

How? Inhale gently through the nose, letting your abdomen swell as much as it will to a slow count of five. Continue to breathe in **through the nose** to another count of five, this time letting your ribs expand under your hands and finally your chest too. Hold your breath for a count of five. Now slowly let it out through your mouth as you count slowly to ten, noticing how your rib cage shrinks and pulling in with your abdomen until you have released all the air. Repeat this exercise 6 times.

We already described at other moments in this work the Deep Breathing techniques. We know it is not to upset you that we repeat it, but because it is one of the cornerstones of your successful transgression. Repetition is the best way to master new information. Remember how you learned your alphabet or your mat tables.

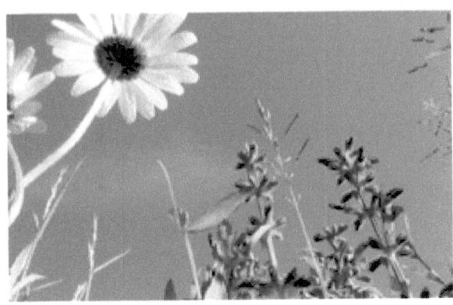

Please do thus your deep breathing exercises consciously and with dedication minimum morning and evening. Ask professional advice and follow a yoga course to learn the technique fully if you have questions about it. Then you will pick up the advantages yourself and you will start telling or teaching people you love and estimate. Children should and can master this breathing from early age as that's what they do automatically the first months of their venue.

"Our bodies are recreating themselves constantly - we, make a skeleton every 3 months, new skin every month. We are capable of reversing the Aging Process!!"
~ Deepak Chopra, *'Magical Mind Magical Body'*

Brain strengthening activities can help you delay or escape memory loss and perhaps Alzheimer's disease. Word puzzles, Sudoku, ... or train your brain at sites as 'aadl.org/node/918' , 'cognitivelabs.com', ...

Full-body exercises and brisk walking will help improve blood and oxygen flow throughout the body, which will keep facial skin looking younger and healthier (anti-wrinkle).

Lets **"C.O.K.E."!**   "COKE" is the **"EnjoyVity"** acronym for **"Car, Office or Kitchen Exercises"**. Make it easier for you to remember. Here are eight (8) of the **"C.O.K.E."**-exercises you should do regularly and can do at any moment (some even unnoticed) within the brackets you find the pages where we talk about them:

Zero neck roll (29)	Smile (101)	Kuhne's Ice Packing (111)
Kegel's / Pubis Squeeze (167)	SOT point (170)	Deep Breath (173)
Einsteins (181)	Yawn (8 & 182)	

Make **"C.O.K.E."** your favorite, do at least 4 per day and rotate through them on a regular basis. Ask yourself every day at 9 PM 'did I fully C.O.K.E.'.
Repetition is key for success. Read and practice over again, get the clear picture in your mind, become a master in **"EnjoyVity"**.

So remember say "No, thank you"
    to shallow breathing

    to endless coach hanging

So remember you can add years to your life

    by 'C.O.K.E.' -ing

    by understanding that Repetition is

    the best way to master your change

14. Live Your dreams

When truth and desire meet, dreams are born. ~*unknown*

Write/think your scenario, believe it and live it

You 'are already' not you 'will once'

Visualize yr day-dreams

In your mind and on paper, pictures, make a scrapbook.
Visualize and dynamize your well thought over and defined goals in life, this is key!
Need help: 'visualizeyourgoals.com' or look at and use the vision board of 'orangepeel.co.nz'

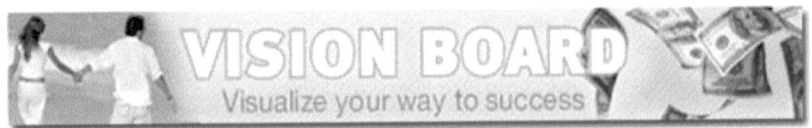

Work at your level

Delegate or avoid and at best refuse what's beyond your competencies

Being close to the top of your 'competencies' leads to stress, acute diseases, ... Being over that top though brings you in a possible free fall with depressions, burn out, chronic diseases, Alzheimer, suicide, ...

Know those limits of your competencies

Use your intuition

How to: settle into a comfortable position, sitting upright. Close your eyes and slowly inhale and exhale, letting your mind gradually quiet down. When thoughts intrude, try not to concentrate on them. Keep focusing on your breath to center yourself. When your mind feels calm, pose a question such as, "What can heal any aches I have?" In the next few moments notice what your intuition says. Just let go, relax. Practice. In time, intuitive answers will come more easily. Is not this Meditation, a pray?

Short-/mid-term revenues, salaries,... should not be your first guideline.
Finances are only a small part of your true wealth
Make a comparison table with your strong- and weak points in relation to that existing or new challenge

> !KEY! Is it or they, or will it or they, give me or bring me 'more' <u>satisfaction?</u>
>
> 'No, no, no' don't become a 'rolling stone' without satisfaction.
>
> Question yourself, your, maybe exotic, goals, your friends, will they still be there if you fail, your lifestyle, do you need that larger house, second car, golf-club-membership, ... , ... is this job, challenge, ..., even hobby fun?
>
> if the answer is no or not really then quit
>
> is it captivating or boring
>
> what was your deepest desire, what you wanted to accomplish in your life, what 'were' your dreams
>
>> did you forget about them/are there non left?
>> Then take a day/week/month/year break and find out!
>
> Re-booth your life, it is never too late
>
>> Take charge
>>
>> only push the 'feel good' buttons you want
>>
>> spend time with or on 'Your' life goals, and less with or on those of others
>>
>> relocate, refresh, return (to your old love/job/village/...)

Avoid long term emotions and stress (put it on your muscles not on your heart, stomach or brain)

> See also chapter 1
>
> It certainly exists that heart surgeons dye from a stroke and that neuro-surgeons pass away with a brain tumor.
>
> How much stress can you get before being tired, exhausted, disappointed, down, depressed, sick, ..., unconscious, irreversibly out of balance, incurable, ...

Serenity is something marvelous, the key to the psychological and physical health. Who is serene, goes without fear and aggression through life, is relaxed and confident. Serenity, simplicity and clarity are the three pillars of a philosophical art of living.

Remain in balance and serene, even if it becomes stormy.
Live simply while concentrating on the substantial.
Be cheerful and able to laugh with oneself and the absurdity of life. Make it fun!

Always keep a buffer (reserve) for unforeseen problems, which you then will be able to confront

- Enjoy all 4 season's, weather is not and will never be an issue for any of your plans

- Touch, smell, listen, feel, taste and contemplate (walk slower, tilt your head slightly to the right and watch to the left and upper side).

Take 'Your' time

- As said with meditation, practicing yoga, sophrology (serenity, harmony and spirit study) or praying you can almost stop the time

- Manage your time

- Get organized

- Clean up your agenda, your desk, clear tasks and your mind.

'Feeling rich' costs nothing and will make you happy right away

Never stop playing

- Keep the child in you vivid

- Laugh daily or at least put a smile on your face its +50% of the and 'your' solution

- How: bring your mouth-corners towards your ears and your eyebrows. Upupup!

- And/or visualize your greatest dream or join a laugh-course

Sleep less but more intensive. Noticed already that you sleep more when depressed than when you are excited and happy to be alive?

You Spend Over a 1/3 of Your Life Sleeping!

6 maximum 8 hours should be enough for most of us! See table

Typical Sleep Needs

Group	Amount of Sleep Needed
Infants	About 16 hours per day of sleep
Babies and toddlers	From 6 months to 3 years: between 10 and 14 hours per day. Infants and young children generally get their sleep from a combination of nighttime sleep and naps.
Children	Ages 3 to 6: between 10 and 12 hours of sleep Ages 6 to 9: about 10 hours of sleep Ages 9 to 12: about 9 hours of sleep
Teenagers	About 9 hours of sleep per night. Teens have trouble getting enough sleep not only because of their busy schedules, but also because they are biologically programmed to want to stay up later and sleep later in the morning, which usually doesn't mesh with school schedules.
Adults	For most adults, 6, 7 to 8 hours a night appears to be the best amount of sleep.
Older adults	Older adults are also thought to need 7-8 hours of sleep. However, this sleep may be for shorter time spans, is lighter than a younger adult's, and may include a nap during the day.
Pregnant women	During pregnancy, women may need a few more hours of sleep per night, or find that they need small catnaps during the day.

So how much sleep do YOU need? A rule of thumb is to consider how you normally feel after sleep. Do you feel refreshed and alert, or groggy and exhausted? If you don't feel refreshed, chances are you're not sleeping enough. If you are falling asleep as soon as your head hits the pillow, regularly need an alarm clock to wake up, or feel the need for frequent naps during the day, it is very likely you are sleep deprived. Sleep requirements are highly individual and depend on many factors:

1. your age and genetic makeup
2. what you do during your waking hours, including exercise
3. the quality of your sleep

There are short sleepers who only need 4 and also a few long sleepers who may need 12, but that is really exceptional. Dr. Gary Feldman (Sleep Basics for Children and Parents)states that **over 47 million American adults are** what is termed **'sleep deprived'**, not getting the 7-8 hours per night they need to function. Sleep deprived, possibly operate with a **diminished IQ, immune system** and a decreased ability to be efficient or effective and impossible to show up as healthy in their relationships. All of which severely impair their ability to be effective, healthy, and happy.

Researchers from the University of Warwick and University College of London have found that lack of sleep can more than double the risk of death from cardiovascular disease, but that too much sleep can also double the risk of death. Short sleep has been shown to be a risk factor for weight gain, hypertension and Type 2 diabetes. An excess of sleep can lead to depression, sloth and mental inactivity—proven obstacles to long life. If you could get closer to **6-8 hours** of sleep a night, you could **add time** to your life. a University of California, San Diego psychiatry study of more than one million adults found that people who live the longest self-report sleeping for six to seven hours each night.

Exercise is key to falling asleep easily and sleeping more deeply. If you have trouble falling asleep exercise more or wake up earlier.

Bring down your sleeping time step by step, by half hour portions for instance, as you are interfering with your **'biological clock'**. Air-transport personal and people who travel across several time zones (jetlag) or rotating shift workers (sleep disorders) know the importance of regularity and stability in the sleep pattern. Light therapy and melatonine supplementation are known remedies. The biological or circadian rhythm is a roughly 24 hour cycle shown by physiological processes in our body. Once you reach your goal you can set your alarm on your minimum wanted sleeping hours whatever the time you go to sleep.

Take care if you are overweight and/or have sleep apnea you should take care of these before or while correcting your sleep pattern.

Not enough or too much! Sleep-specialists consider that for adults 'uninterruptedly' sleeping between **6.5 and 7.5 hours** is enough and will be guided by your biological watch. You should listen to your biological watch and as such keep her and your sleeping time in balance. The extended studies of professor Kripke (1979) showed that less than 25% had the above mentioned optimal sleeping time and that over 45% of Americans slept between 8 and 9 hours and close to 10% even more than 9 hours.

"The major mortality risk associated with habitual sleep duration is among long sleepers, by which I mean those sleeping eight hours or more." Daniel F. Kripke, MD, Professor of Psychiatry at the University of California, San Diego

A recent survey by the American Cancer Society found that participants who slept an average of **seven hours** a day had the lowest mortality rates.

Shigeaki Hinohara, known physician, from now +97, sleeps 6 hours a day and states:" **Energy comes from feeling good, not from eating or sleeping a lot."**

An optimum sleep pattern can add many months even many years to your life:

Added conscious years in function of hrs of less sleep/night and expected remaining life expectancy (ERLE)

3hr/night less	1,25	2,5	3,12	3,7	5	6,2	7,5	8,75	10	11,25	12,5
2hr/night less	0,83	1,66	2	2,5	3,32	4	5	5,8	6,6	7,5	8,32
1hr/night less	0,41	0,83	1	1,25	1,66	2	2,5	2,9	3,3	3,75	4,16
ERLE		10	20	**25**	30	40	50	60	70	80	90	100

Example 1: if you are now 55 and your normal life expectancy is 80 you can add to the **25 years left** an extra '**one (1) very conscious year**' by just sleeping on average one hour less per night. Thus you add 1 full attentive year 'within' your life by sleeping on average 7 instead of 8 hours. It is all in your mind!

Example 2: if you are only 20 today then for sure with the right approach and 21st century life enhancement technologies you will make it another healthy *80* years till you are 1-hundred. Bringing your true 'sleep-span' down from 9 to 6 hours will create you an extra '*10 attentive years*'!

What you say? Choose your healthy sleep- path and enjoy the gained extra months and years. Use these extra quarters or even hours for YOUR self-development.

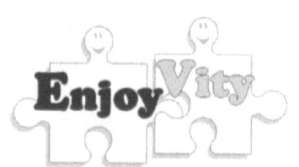

Your Full Spectrum of Life

Snoring:

Avoid your bedmate's nightmare! Stop snoring for both partner's sake. By constriction of the air-path the air flow will tremble at breathing, this can lead to snoring. People who snore often have too much throat and nasal tissue, or "floppy" tissue that is more prone to vibrate. There are many reasons which lead to snoring an important one can be the elongation or relaxation of the palate. Snoring occurs on all ages but increases with the age by a bulge of the mucous membrane in the pharynx by an increase of fat

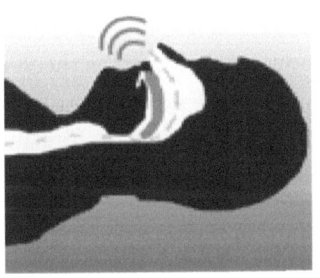

tissue and by a softening of mucous membrane and skin. Ask for medical advice first, as there are many techniques and solutions available as well. Or inform about the 'white noise machine' it creates a consistent, smooth sound of rushing air to help control unwanted intermittent or continuous noise, such as traffic, nearby conversation and yes snoring.

Free of charge and natural actions to reinforce your uvula area: just play trumpet or hobo or pretend to play while in- and exhaling with short puffs (increases also lung capacity, remember), put on a Einstein-like, Polynesian dancer or lion face (*), sing your known children's song as ie, ie, ie, or ho, ho , ho or make the sound "ung-

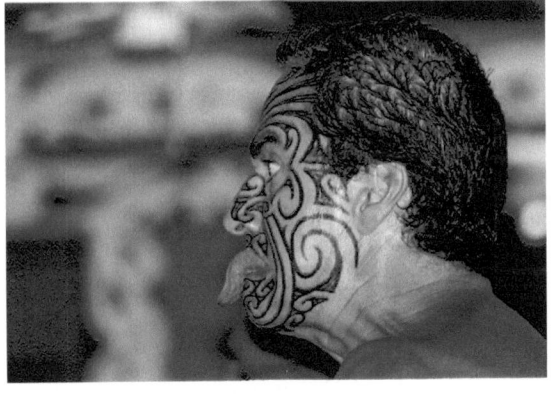

gah" repetitively ; for details read and practice Dr. Elizabeth Scott's 'the natural way to stop snoring' or Alice Ojay's 'Singing for Snorers': 'singingforsnorers.com'.

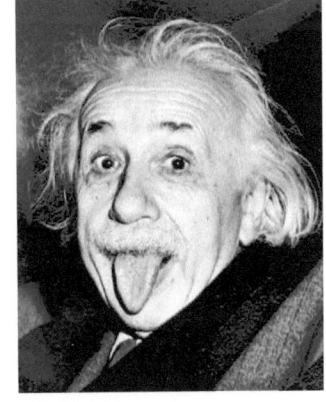

(*) eyebrows up, mouth angles towards your ears, tongue out reaching for your chin; repeat 6 times min 3 times/day.
Also great taking distance of over-serious daily routines: DESTRESS!

Snoring can turn into **sleep apnea** which leads to very serious health risks. Get informed and find medical help especially if mentioned exercises together with improved eating-, drinking- and moving habits do not bring serious relief in 6 weeks.

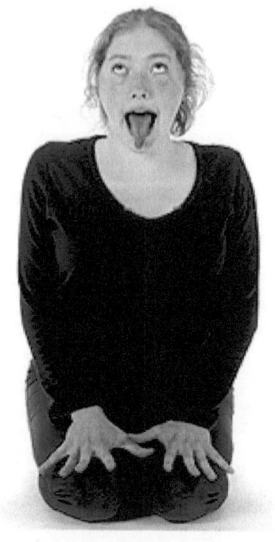

Hatha-Yogi know this 'grimace' as the *Simha-asana*, the lion pose, the **destroyer of all diseases**. Simhasana gives stretch to face and arms and relieves tension in the chest and face. Posture: Sit up on the knees (or on a chair), hands on the knees, keep the back erect, inhale while stretching the mouth the jaws as wide as possible, extend the tongue out and downward as much as possible, fix your gaze either at the tip of the nose or between the eyebrows and stretch the fingers straight out from the knees. Hold the posture for the duration of the inhaled breath then exhale, dropping the fingers to the knees and closing the mouth and eyes. The same grimace/exercise pops-up in 21st century buzz called **'face-yoga'**: with face-specific exercises formulated to combat wrinkles through relaxation and tension reduction, and to tone the muscles as a preventive measure.

Hold the *simha-asana* for thirty to sixty seconds and repeat three to five times. Go roaring loadly like a lion as you enter into the 'Lion Pose' while sticking your tongue out. This stimulates the throat and cultivates courage and fearlessness.

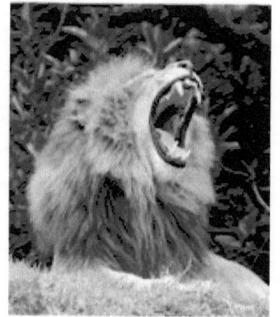

An easy way to **fake yawning** over and over again... that relaxes and completely opens up the throat: sit comfortably, close your eyes, loose that lower jaw, breath in from your stomach (should feel your diaphragm move), press with your tongue-tip continuously the front of your palate, breath out ... and repeat 6 times. You will start yawning thoroughly, let it happen and repeat the exercise; it's good to strengthen your palate and throat tissue while it further also relaxes you. This exercise is also part of the relaxation practice exercise; see Chapter 10. About 'fast reading'!

Be prepared to sleep well and have great dreams.

Use the right pillows, cushions, covers and a healthy mattress.
Does your bed to be headed in a certain direction? East or South?

"Never lie down to sleep with your head northward or westward" is a common injunction given from time immemorial by the Indian mother to her children. Almost every Hindu- orthodox or heterodox- observes this dictum of his ancestors, but he doesn't know the rationale or significance behind the dictum, although it has been handed down to him through generations. This applies only to the inhabitants of the Northern Hemisphere. The inhabitants of the Southern Hemisphere must lay down their bodies with head northward.   While the Chinese **Feng Shui** states: don't turn the head to the West because that is the direction that all human souls are traveling to.
South or East seem thus to be the best bed-head direction in the Northern hemisphere. The 'bed-head' direction is one of the very first factors to think about while designing your house or apartment and before you put in other furnish into your bedroom as it can influence your sleep comfort.

If you remain with undeclared effects or strange situations, you can also have your sleeping place checked-out against geopathic stress and/or electro-stress by means of a radiestesic- or dowsing-specialist. Remember, everything in the Universe vibrates with a definite frequency and our cells, organs and body can be influenced by electro-smog and other unforeseen frequencies.

If you have questions about electromagnetic field, microwave radiation health and related very actual topics, the like mobile phones and WiFi, read also page 83 and check-out: 'powerwatch.org.uk'.

Sleep in a 'DARK' bedroom: +95% darkness or put eye-covers

Sleep in a 'QUIET' bedroom: maximum 30dBA or put earplugs

Know and use your sleep rituals, calm down, tea, forget about others problems, read some poems, deep breath, touch your 'sea of tranquility' (page 170), 'zero-neck-roll', ...

Learn to dream

We dream in color during what is called the REM (rapid eye movement) sleep. You will have 3 to 5 REM sleeps per night. Your body is paralyzed, but no matter what a dream is about, REM sleep will cause an erection in a man who is not impotent.

There's a reason you dream at night. It's NOT random nonsense. When you are dreaming you are thinking on a much deeper, more focused and insightful level than when you're awake. When you're dreaming you're actually problem solving... it's just in a different language.   Lauri Quinn Loewenberg, dream expert as seen on popular TV programs such as The View, Good Morning America, Anderson Cooper 360, The Today Show and on a CNN special "Sleep with Dr. Sanjay Gupta."

How much dreams I had then so far? Check it out: 'thedreamzone.com'

See also chapter 9 about 'be creative exercise' (brain stimulation)

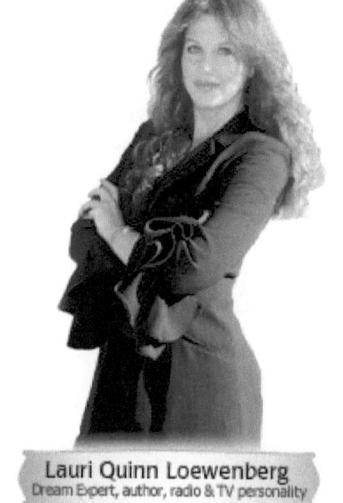
Lauri Quinn Loewenberg
Dream Expert, author, radio & TV personality

We dream every 90 minutes during the **REM** stage of sleep. But dreams aren't captured by the intellect; you need intuition to grasp them. Pay attention to your dreams. You may be surprised at the practical advice they offer, such as tips on romance and job stress. By initiating a dialogue with your dreams, you can receive ingenious solutions to your questions and problems. You will have an increased knowledge about yourself, bring about self-awareness and self-healing. Dreams can help guide you through difficult decisions, relationship issues, health concerns, career questions or any life struggle you may be going through.

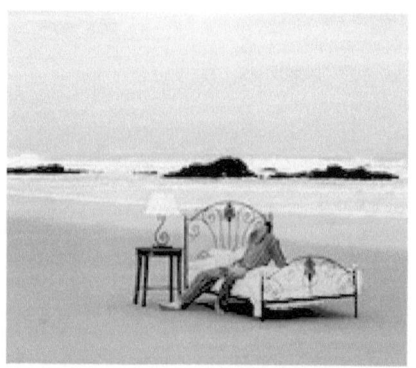

Lucid Dreaming: as we learned earlier the average person spends 8 hours a day sleeping, and lives an average life of about +75 years, then he or she has slept nearly 25 years of her life away.

Can we get more out of all those years than just rest? For sure it is a language and skill you can learn to understand. It is fun once managed. Be aware and learn about conscious dreaming. Once you are aware you are dreaming you can alter your dreams and dictate what happens: you can do anything you've ever wanted, go anywhere you've ever desired! 'dreamviews.com'

Get your FREE introduction at 'dreammanifesto.com' and check: 'dreammoods.com'.

Recalling Your Dreams : Before going to bed, tell yourself that : "I will remember my dream when I wake up". Pose one specific question, as, "Is this project right for me? Keep a pencil/notebook next to your bed so that it will be within reach as soon as you wake up and you can jot them down before they slip away. Upon waking from a dream, lay still in your bed, keeping your eyes closed and moving as little as possible. Wake up slowly and stay relaxed. Hold on to the feelings you have and let your mind wander to the images of what you have just dreamt. Were you frustrated, terrified, or happy? Write down as many details in your dream as you can, no matter how minute or seemingly unimportant it may be. Do not judge the content or worry if it makes sense. The idea is to get it down on paper so you can evaluate it later. Sometimes it may help to draw pictures. Learn to share your dreams and talk about them with others, no matter who seemingly insignificant. The more often you acknowledge your dreams and bring them into "reality", the easier it will be to remember them.

Because you are still awake not dreaming but reading, find out about ...

The Sixth Great Extinction: Human beings (that is you and me, not others only) are currently causing the greatest mass extinction of species since the extinction of the dinosaurs 65 million years ago. If present trends continue **one half of all species of life** on earth will be extinct in less than 100 years (~E. O. Wilson of Harvard, the world's most esteemed biologist), as a result of habitat destruction, pollution, invasive species, and climate change.

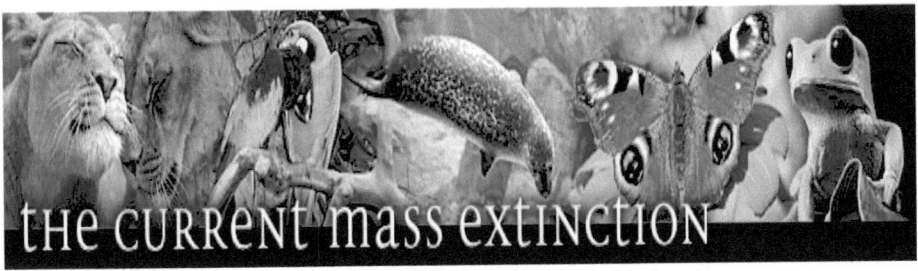

Lets give David Ulansey and his world wide team an **urgent** hand 'well.com'; read *'Rewilding North America'* by Dave Foreman or find an introduction 'rewilding.org'. Lazy to read, then please just listen at 'well.com' to Prof. Ulansey's audio. Yes it is that important for you and your posterity.

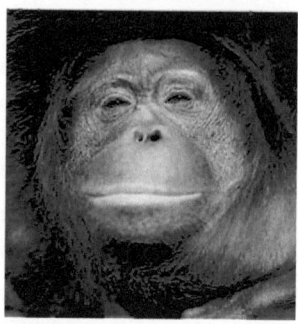

They *all* thank you already.

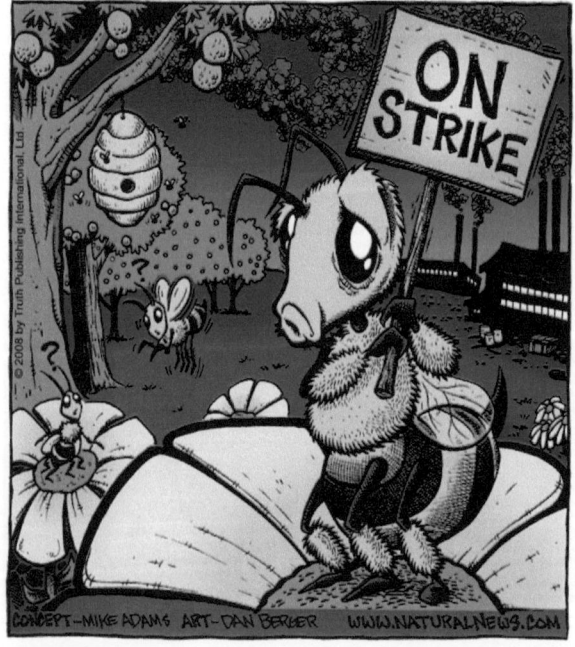

Honeybees are disappearing massively by CCD (colony collapse disorder) .Honeybees pollinate 130 different crops, which supply $15 billion worth of food and ingredients each year. One out of every three bites of food on your dinner plate was made possible by honeybee pollination. In general, human beings have a very poor appreciation of all the services "provided" by Mother Nature, including the removal of CO_2 from the air by plants, the turning of soil by worms, and of course the free pollination of crops and orchards by honeybees and other insects. Read more: 'naturalnews.com' . Bee populations are vulnerable to pesticides, but what about genetically modified crops or factors such as the recent increase in atmospheric electromagnetic radiation as a result of growing numbers of cell phones and wireless communication towers. Follow this issue and take action, it is about your and our children's survival 'organicconsumers.org' and 'vanishingbees.co.uk/'.

Largest and oldest collective apiary in the world at Inzerki/Ida ou Ziki/Sousse/Morocco
The 'Taddart Ouguerram' apiary is hidden on a Southern slope at 980 meters height in a very rich green eco-environment and holds over 300 beehives and this within living memory. *So there was a healthy social and sweet live also before our refined white sugar decades.* It **needs restoration** after recent inundation; the neighboring area is also called the 'paradise valley': 'visitmorocco.com'

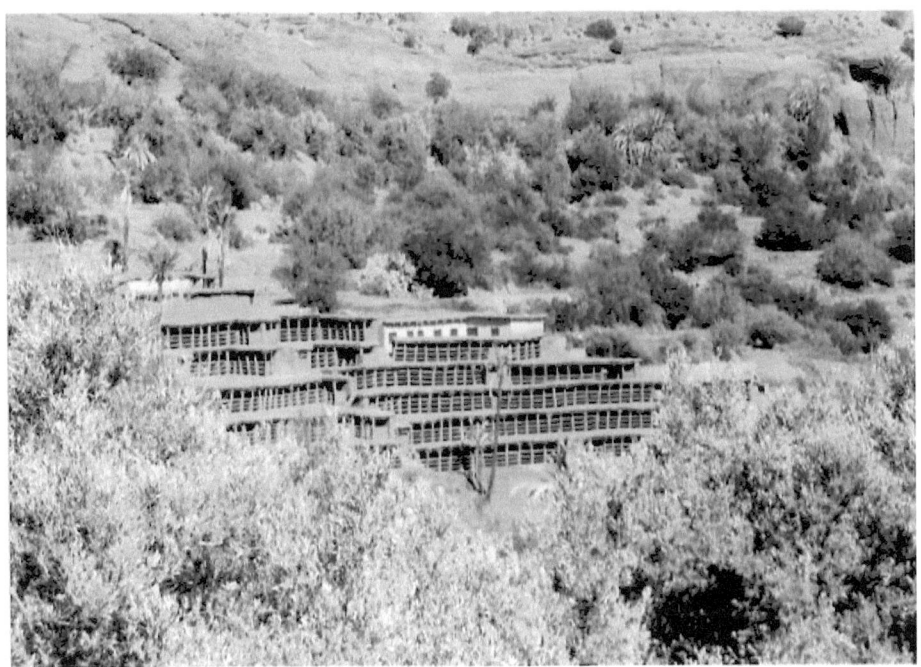

"What I note, are the current devastations, the alarming disappearance of the living species, whether plant or animal; and due to its current density, mankind lives under a kind of mode of 'internal poisoning' – so to speak - and I think of the present and the world in which I am finishing my existence. This n' is not a world that I like." ~ Claude Lévi-Strauss, anthropologist, born 28 November 1908; died 30 October 2009.

Yes, we have to change our way of living, eating, behaving! WE have to change our world as WE are in charge. Get informed and motivated, watch the movie-trailer: 'we-feed-the-world.at'

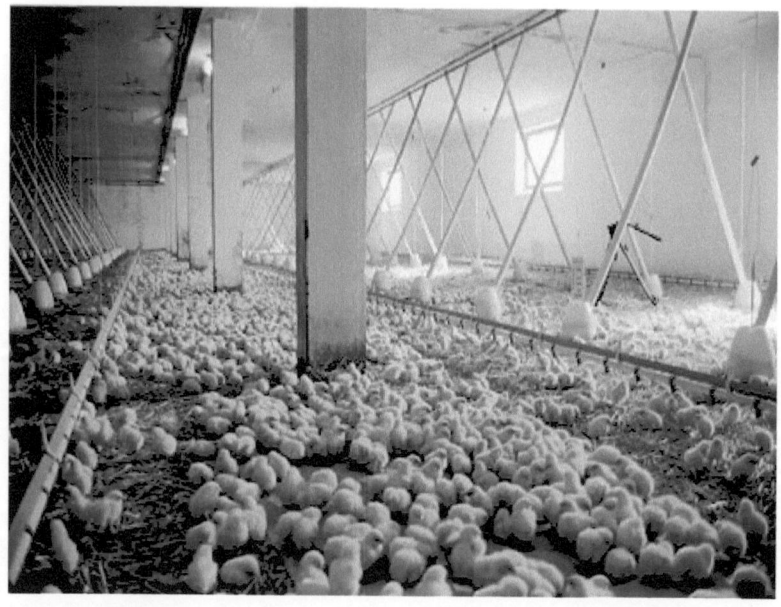

So remember say "No, thank you"
> to nonchalance

> to under- or oversleeping

> to snoring

So remember you can add years to your life
> by only living 'Your' dreams

> by self-controlling the choices of your future

> by taking action for a better You which always leads to a better less stressed world, you then can ***enjoy*** to live on even longer

15. Create your paradise

> "Life is not measured by the number of breaths we take,
> but by the moments that take our breath away." ~ unknown

Do it 'now' not in another life.

The big faiths of mankind should be brought in harmony with modern scientific evolutionary discoveries. Understand and maybe accept your religious misformation, but certainly study actual science and read inspiring works as "the God delusion" by Richard Dawkins or "Worlds in Collision" by Immanuel Velikovsky or "Shajara Code, Decoded" by Imad Hassan before dogmatizing, not to say contaminating your offspring with complexes. How can you be sure that the faith given at your birth is the only true one? Well then don't limit the horizons of your children, don't traumatize them, don't abuse their minds, let history not repeat itself over and over. Religious choices if any should be taken by individuals once they were able to concert and evaluate the total pallet of choices.

"For universal peace, mankind should agree that ignorance is our shared enemy and that we should all unite to fight, instead of fighting each other over insignificant differences!"Dr Imad Hassan

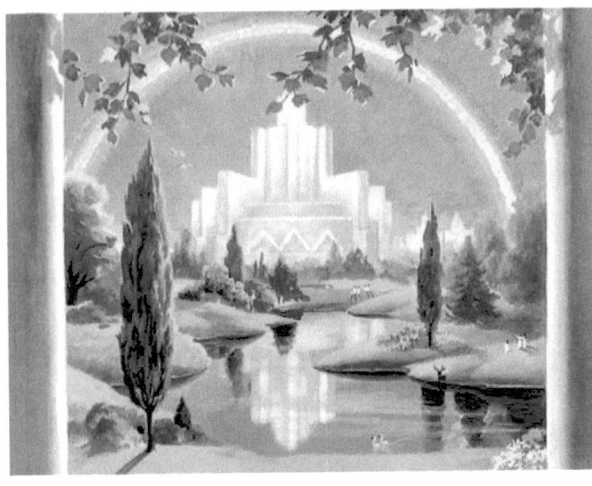

Hence 'Paradise' is for people who reflect!

Paradise: Its not about tropical trees and weather but about 'you' in balance in life and that can be anywhere in the world. Just imagine!

"In the shoreless ocean of reality, man finds only what he seeks"
~ Dr Alexis Carrel, Nobel Prize winner

In earth's atmosphere, raindrops disperse light forming rainbows.
In our energetic world, mind drops disperse towards your full life spectrum.

PARADISE

Your Full Spectrum of Life

Live on a hill, have a 360 degree vision and view

Keep your 'low' profile high

Develop your memory (do the Dennison's, practice fast-read, brainpower,...pages 139, 144 & 136)

Create your 'positive' network, stick with the enthusiast, the trustful, the original, the builders of a better world, thus the genuine, the best.

It is all energy and in 'your' mind.

Be your own artist, play music, draw, paint, write, photograph, ... Also live like an artist, contemplate and become +80 for sure

Find your balance

>Keep perspective, question yourself regularly

>Appreciate nature to its full extend. Go hiking, wildwater fishing or birdwatch ing rather than hunting or golfing. Bring variation in your pass times.

>Dance, sing, meditate, and watch flowers, animals, stars, ... daily and whistle with Toots (Tielemans) your 'bluesette' , it is easy ('lastfm.fr')

Feast regularly, invite, travel, explore different cultures, get and stay in touch. Learn, re-invest, rediscover yourself and grow into your paradise.

Listen, contemplate, enjoy.

"Brand" your own name! Believe in yourself, thus love yourself first.

>Know your roots, research your family's history, build your genealogy tree: 'familytreemaker.com'

Be your own life coach or find one, which will teach you stress management as well as time management prioritizing and goal setting, health maintenance and other life-enhancing habits. Read also page 99.

Learn to say: YES, Thank You!

> Whenever you catch your 'Paradise second, minute ....moment'.

So remember say "No, thank you"
> **to dogma's**
>
> **to ignorance**

So remember you can add years to your life
> **by having a 360° view**
>
> **by finding your balance**

16. My golden age, up to and over 100

"Man today is structured and has natural and pharmacological means in order to arrive till 120 years" ~ Prof. Carlo Vergani, Director of the Geriatrics and Gerontology chair, University of Milan

History of average life expectancy (longevity) from biblical times till today

Variation over time: Humans live on average 31.99 years in Swaziland and on average 82 years in Japan (2008 est.). The oldest confirmed recorded age for any human is 122 years, though some people are reported to have lived longer. Although there are several longevity myths mostly in different stories that were spread in some cultures, there is no scientific evidence of a human living for hundreds of years at any point of time. The following information is derived from the *Encyclopaedia Britannica*, 1961, as well as other sources:

Humans by Era	Average Lifespan at Birth (years)	Comment
Upper Paleolithic	33	At age 15: 39 (thus to age 54)
Neolithic	20	
Bronze Age	18	
Classical Greece	20-30	
Classical Rome	20-30	
Pre-Columbian North America	25-35	
Medieval Islamic Caliphate	35+	The average lifespans of the scholarly class were 59–84.3 years in the Middle East and 69–75 in Islamic Spain.
Medieval Britain	20-30	
Early 20th Century	30-40	
Current world average	66.12 (2008 est.)	~source wikipedia.org

Actual life expectancy

20th century: "Riley is quite correct in assuming that in the years since 1910, among the fifteen percent of the world's population who live in the West and are not members of marginalized social groupings, life expectancy has risen dramatically. In these privileged regions (North America, West Europe, Australia and Japan), by the end of the twentieth century the majority of women could expect to live into their mid-eighties and the majority of men into their late seventies. And in a few selected corners of the non-West such as Costa Rica, Cuba and Kerala State in India, the percentage of people over the age of sixty actually found in regional communities was beginning to resemble the situation found in the West." Rising Life Expectancy: A Global History. ~ James C. Riley, Cambridge University Press, New York 2001.

21st century: Populations are aging worldwide. This means that people are living longer, and the number of older persons is increasing. These trends are evident in American society, as well as in many countries around the world. In the U.S., of those born in 1900 nearly half died before they were 50 years old. People born today can expect to live beyond their 75th year. In 1900 about one in 25 Americans was over 65; today one in eight is over 65. And the age group growing fastest in our society and in many other countries is the "very old," people aged 85 and over. The growth of the elderly population will continue into the future. By the middle of the 21st century, one in five Americans will be over 65, and there will be 15 to **18 million persons over the age of 85**. Dixit the Gerontological Society of America

Record: Life expectancy average is 81,1 years (84,5 for women and 77,7 for men) in **Sardinia**, it shares with the Japanese island of Okinawa, the highest rate of centenarians in the world, among its population (22 centenarians/100.000 inhabitants and 33 centenarians/100.000 Okinawans).

US demographic statistics

- 0 –19 years: 27.4%   (male 42,667,761; female 40,328,895)
- 20–64 years: 60.1%   (male 89,881,041; female 90,813,578)
- 65 years and over: 12.6% (male 15,858,477; female 21,991,195)

US Population projections   (2008 US Census Bureau data)

- 2010: 310,232,863
- 2020: 341,386,665
- 2030: 373,503,674
- 2040: 405,655,295
- 2050: 439,010,253

US Life expectancy (*source:* Census Bureau, 2007):

- total population: 78.10 years
- male: 75.20 years
- female: 81.00 years

Europe (the EU countries) has a population of roughly 499 million. Non-EU countries situated in Europe in their entirety account for another 101 million. Five transcontinental countries have a total of 240 million people, of which about half reside in Europe proper. The largest ethnic groups of Europe are the Russians (with some 90 million settling in the European parts of Russia), followed by the Germans (76 million), French (63 million), Italians (58 million), English (45 million), Spanish (42 million), Poles (42 million) and the Ukrainians (41 million). The total European population will rather stabilize or decrease towards 2050. Europe has 30-40 major languages depending on definition.

Life expectancy West-Europe (*source:* EHEMU, 2003):

- total population: 78.78 years
- male: 75.97 years
- female: 81.60 years

More figures on health, obese and aging in chapter 25 of the book.

Give blood! A **hypothesis** why woman live **+5 years** longer than men, could be due to menstruation, which can cause iron deficiency over a large part of a woman's life. Interestingly, men who donate blood regularly experience the same longevity as women.

If after reading part, most or all of the here set out information you agree that the "**Enjoy**Vity" approach is doable, holistic and the one to spread, than do so.

Send the FREE introduction to a friend... 'enjoyvity.com/linksender/link.php'

If, for the WHO, old age is "65 years and more", the seniors do not feel old at 60 years and with progress of medicine, they hope neither to feel as such at 70 years. Being 50 years, an individual can from now on hope to live still 35 years and thus did not achieve half of its adult. The great age (or physiological decline) does not start nowadays, except disease, before 75 years.

Many signs of the ageing which we allot to age are actually ascribable to some extent with our excesses: tobacco, excess of sun, bad food, stress, lack of exercise...

Do understand that aging is mainly the loss of electrons with oxidation as result.

Hence the lifespan of our body and tissue can be expanded by minimizing oxidation through reduction with healthy foods, drinks, lifestyle,... and correct medical 'reducing' responses. As in the 21st century we should finally accept that our life functions are primarily controlled by physics.

Healthy till 80+ for sure

You are designed and built to last over a century why settle for less

Aging, particularly aging well and staying healthy, is increasingly a hot topic as the population grays, people live longer and tens of millions of baby-boomers enter or approach their 60s.

Take the Eons Longevity Calculator at 'eons.com/calculator' and cheer up. The online 'Eons' community for baby boomers, has partnered with Tom Perls, a physician and leading researcher in the study of aging at Boston University School of Medicine, to develop its Longevity Calculator. The 10-minute survey, which is available for free, uses information you submit about your health, lifestyle, and family history to tell you how long you might live. It also provides a personalized "To-Do" list for you and your physician. More also at Dr. Perls related website 'livingto100.com'.

Follow at 'longevitymeme.org/newsletter' the latest on news, opinions and commentary for people interested in healthy life extension: making use of diet, lifestyle choices, technology and proven medical advances to live longer, healthier lives, links to interesting resources and more.

'Anti-aging': the last decade a fully buzzed magic, hyper-word. The **anti-aging** science addresses how to prevent, slow, or reverse the effects of aging and help people live longer, healthier and happier lives.   The 'EnjoyVity' themes are clearly integrated in the 'life extension' expectations of all of us, but in a balanced holistic way assuring improved health and quality of life for all those and at any age who respect its basic, simple and easy to follow, as still genetically imprinted, rules. Aging in good health is **a lifelong task**.

Orthomolecular therapy offers selective supplementation of vitamins and other nutrients that are essential to delay the aging process. They include vitamins C, D and E, coenzyme Q10, selenium, alpha-lipoic acid, chromium, folic-acid, L-carnitine, quercetin and others. Two-time Nobel Prize winner, and molecular biologist,

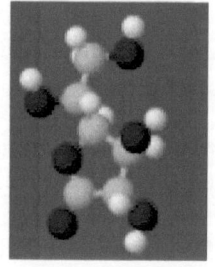

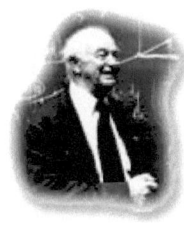
Linus Pauling, Ph.D.,coined the term "Orthomolecular" in 1968. You definitely shouldn't do megadose vitamin therapy without consulting a competent professional first. Find out about an 'OM' practitioner in your area or any nutrient value: 'orthomolecular.org/nutrients'.

Keep your design: look well after your figure and treat it from the
- **inside** with the right foods, drinks, emotions and movements
- **outside** with anti-wrinkle exercises (chapter 7), support of modern cosmetology and when needed why not with little esthetic chirurgic help. *"Americans are obsessed with discovering the fountain of youth. Americans spent a whopping $11.5 billion on cosmetic procedures in 2006"* ~ the American Society of Plastic Surgeons,

Stay artistically independent, flexible, creative and inventive.

Keep it up even when you are down

Learn to say: YES, Thank You!

When starting a brand new day

&

When finishing your beautiful day

to its

Full spectrum.

So remember say "No, thank you"
    to feeling old

    to rigidity

So remember you can add years to your life

    by following the "**Enjoy**Vity" suggestions

    by Giving blood if you are male

And also a "YES, thank you" for making your
    "*C.O.K.E.*'s"

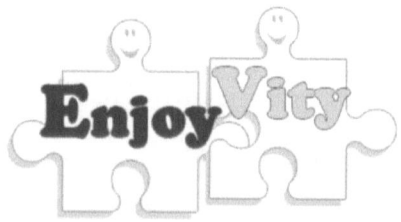

Your Full Spectrum of Life

17. the 7 basic **Enjoy**Vity rules

1. Follow your intuition

2. Laugh (everyday and from the belly)

3. Keep perspective (look at it from outside our globe, galaxy or our universe)

4. Less is much more (eat less and live healthy till +100). Water, fruit and veggies your stable base

5. Exercise but also relax properly

6. Have always dreams and never stop believing in them

7. No time for –isme's (leads to disease)

18. My Personal Full Spectrum

Yes, I want to improve my wellbeing and start living in joy and health till I am over a century old!

Therefore I will keep my biological, emotional and physical **terrain in balance** as shown by the "**Enjoy**Vity®" spirit and approach.

My **biological terrain** will be improved and stay balanced while I eat moderately and a variety of whole, fiber rich, organic, raw, fermented, ... foods which I chew and grind correctly in order to optimize and respect my assimilation and metabolism. Further I will drink a sufficient quantity of low mineral content, pure water with preferably slightly acidic and reduced parameters and I understand about the value of herbal infusions, limited consumption of red wine and champagne. I'll get a detox-cure once a year or when my body tells me.

My **emotional terrain** will be improved while thinking positively, controlling stress, saying 'no thank you', smiling, practice deep breathing and yoga or other mind setting practices. I also empower my socio-cultural contacts, help others, love myself and stay focused on my personal dreams. While feeling happy.

My **physical terrain** will be improved while I eat and drink correctly, move, walk in nature, exercise, tai-chi, **C.O.K.E.** and behave consciously.

For my actual personal calculation I use the average life expectancy figure in my country of 76 for men and 81 for women (see table chapter 25)

I use now the Life Expectancy calculator of Dr.Perls at 'livingto100.com', or through the 'eons' site at 'eons.com/calculator' which will calculate my real theoretical life duration and which might be lower or higher than the above average figure.

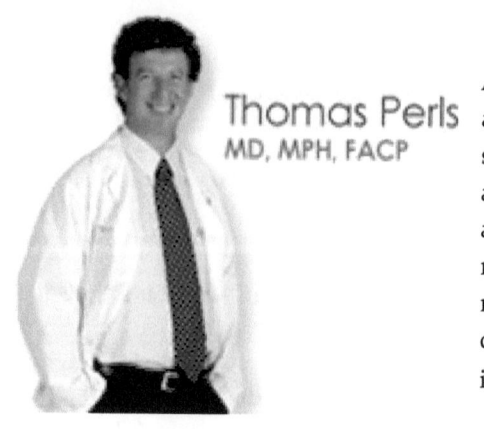

Thomas Perls
MD, MPH, FACP

Also will I find out about my personal adjustments to make, taking in account stress management, brain strengthening and stimulation, working hours management and a positive attitude. Minimizing UV-exposure, caffeine intake, red meat, fast food, sweets,..., as also clearly brought to my attention by the insides of the "**Enjoy** Vity" approach.

I can also take and read the detailed longevity test based on D.Woodruff -Pak Ph.D. studies at 'enjoyvity.com/ longevity_quiz.pdf'.

I will as such extend my life with many EXTRA "'**Enjoy** Vitalic" years and months beyond my actual life expectancy.

I can thus look out to still **enjoy** my days while being over 90 years.

My personal result: ....

Taking in account ...., ...,........................, ..., ...
and........................ as brought to me by the insides of this "**Enjoy** Vity" book, I will extend my life with ..... years and .... months.

So I remember and am saying

"YES, thank you"

to myself for understanding that change

is here and now,

but by me and for me only

So I remember and am saying

"YES, thank you"

to myself for acting holistically

in order to "**Enjoy**" and with full "Vity"

every extra year, month, day and hour of

my wonderful and exclusive life

on this beautiful blue planet in

this dynamic universe.

19. Inspiring Quotes and readings

Mind is everything: muscle, pieces of rubber. All that I am, I am because of my mind. ~Paavo Nurmi

Champions are made from something they have deep inside them - a desire, a dream, a vision. Mahummad Ali

There are only two ways to live your life.
One is as though nothing is a miracle.
The other is as though everything is a miracle.   Albert Einstein

It is thus always possible to speak, even though that leaves from the shadow the lost truths, which will call into question certain scientific concepts built into dogmas by the news. ~ Jeanne Rousseau

I am convinced that life is 10% what happens to me and 90% how I react to it." ~Charles Swindoll

Nothing is a waste of time if you use the experience wisely. ~ Rodin

We humans are the only animal abusing nature since some centuries. ~Yves Verheyen

You must be the change you wish to see in the world. ~ Mahatma Gandhi.

"In the shoreless ocean of reality, man finds only what he seeks"
Dr & Nobel Price winner Alexis Carrel

In order to change we must be sick and tired of being sick and tired.
~Author Unknown

Men for the sake of getting a living forget to live. ~Margaret Fuller

If your dog is fat, you're not getting enough exercise. ~Author Unknown

I want to be thoroughly used up when I die.
For the harder I work, the more I live. ~G.B.Shaw

Desire causes your pain. ~Buddha

"Each morning we are born again. What we do today is what matters most." ~ *Buddha*

" The miracle is this - the more we share, the more we have." ~ Leonard Nimoy

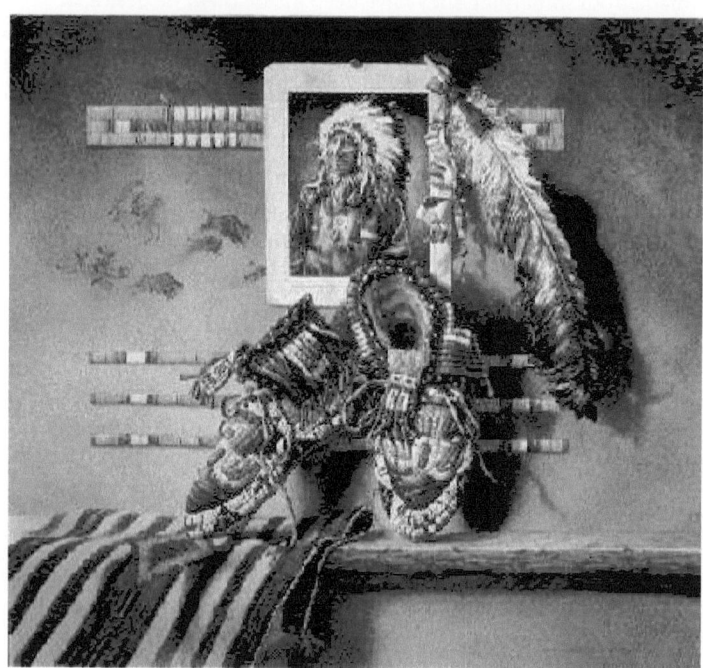

Treat the earth well: it was not given to you by your parents, it was loaned to you by your children. We do not inherit the Earth from our Ancestors, we borrow it from our Children."
Ancient Indian Proverb

Recommended readings and Links

Chopra Deepak *Quantum Healing.* Bantam Books, 1989
Chu Valentin *The yin-yang butterfly.* Putnam's, NY
Dawkins Richard *the God Delusion.* Bantam Press, London, 2006
Dean Sheldon *New Life through natural methods.* New Life Publishing, AZ, 1980
de Bonvoisin Ariane *the First 30 days.* HarperCollins, NY, 2008
De Zutter Andre *Doctor Nature Heals.* Lulu, 2010
Dooley Mike *Notes from the Universe,* 2004
Evans Simon *Brain Fitness.* The brain Code 2007
Finch *The Biology of Human Longevity: Inflammation, Nutrition, and Aging in the Evolution of Lifespans* -2007
Fuller Buckminster *Grunch of Giants,* 1984

Hassan Imad *Shajara Code Decoded*, for the wider benefit of mankind. Authorhouse UK, 2007
Hawking Stephen *A brief History of Time*. Bantans Press, NY 1988
Hay Louise *Heal your body*. Hay House, CA, 1982
Ignarro Louis *NO more heart disease*. St.Martin's Press, NY 2005
Jablonski Nina *Skin: A Natural History,* UC Press 2006
Kuhne Louis : *La Nouvelle Science de guérir* - Leipzig, 1893 – re-edited « La Vie Claire »
Kimbrell Andrew & Co. *'Fatal Harvest'*, Island Press 2002
Perls T.Thomas, Margery Hutter Silver. *Living to 100*, Basic Books 1999
Ojay Alice 'singingforsnorers.com'
Ototake Hirotada, *No One's perfect* -Kodansha International 2000
Scott Elizabeth *The natural way to stop snoring*. Orion Books, London, 1995
Tenpenny Sherry *Saying No to Vaccines: A Resource Guide for All Ages*. NMA media Press 2008
Velikovsky Immanuel *Worlds in Collision*, Doubleday NY 1950
Woodruff Diana *Can you live to be 100?* Chatham Square Press, NY, 1981

www.infoaging.org	American Federation of Aging Research
www.powerwatch.org.uk	Electromagnetic Field and Microwave Radiation health debate
www.oirf.com	Biological Medicine Resource
www.storyofstuff.com	Sustainable Production & Consumption
www.trendsresearch.com	Worldwide Forecasting
www.originalquinton.com	Therapeutic Plasma
www.ourplanet.com	Environment and Development
www.howtobehappy.org	Have Fun Changing the World
www.helpguide.org	Prevent & Resolve Life's challenges
www.ehow.com	How to do about Everything
www.holisticonline.com	Information on your health through conventional, alternative, integrative, and mind-body medicine
www.solveyourproblem.com	You can do it

www.resourcesforlife.com	Resources for Better Living
www.dsc.discovery.com	Taste the Adventure
www.exploratorium.edu	Museum of Science, Art and Human Perception
www.whfoods.com	Healthiest foods
www.bevincent.com	Association Bio-Electronique Vincent
www.mercola.com	Natural Health News
www.nutralegacy.com	Healthy Lifestyle Blog
www.bodyecology.com	Rebuild immunity
www.laleva.org/eng	Hidden Truths
www.earthclinic.com	Folk Remedies
www.cdc.gov/nccdphp/	

20. Acknowledgments and accountability

Useful sources of health advice

This section lists organizations, websites, books and journals which can be useful sources of reliable health information.

Evidence-based healthcare sites for consumers and healthcare providers

- Ottawa Decision Aid Inventory
- Sydney Health Decision Group
- DISCERN
- DiPEx
- Informed Health Online
- Medline Plus
- National Centre for Complementary and Alternative Medicine
- Best Treatments
- National Library for Health (UK)
- Health Insite
- www.wosaam.org world society of anti aging medicine

General government health departments and other official organisations

- National Health Service (NHS)
- National Institute for Health and Clinical Excellence
- National Health & Medical Research Council
- Department of Health and Ageing, Australian Government
- New Zealand Guidelines Group
- Agency for Healthcare Research and Quality
- Travel and vaccine advice - Centers for Disease Control and Prevention

Media

- MediaDoctor (Australia, Canada)
- ABC Radio's Health Report (Australia)
- The New York Times Health Section
- BBC Health Section

More Good addresses throughout the world

Europe

- Alzheimer Scotland - Action on Dementia • Alzheimer's Society • Anchor Trust • Association of Retired and Persons over 50 • The Beth Johnson Foundation • Better Government for Older People • British Association for Service to the Elderly • British Geriatrics Society • British Society of Gerontology • British Society for Research on Ageing • CareUK.net • Centre for Economic Research on Ageing • Centre for Policy on Ageing • Centre for Social Policy Research and Development, University of Wales, Bangor • Dementia Web • DesignAge • English Longitudinal Study of Ageing (ELSA) • European Research Area in Ageing (ERA-AGE) [University of Sheffield] • http://www.healthyageing.nu • IndependentAge (RUKBA) • International Longevity Centre – UK • Keele Centre for Social Gerontology • King's College Institute of Gerontology, London (formerly ACIOG) • The Life Academy • NIACE, Older and Bolder • New Dynamics of Ageing • Oxford Institute of Ageing • Research into Ageing • Third Age Press • U3A, The Third Age Trust, University of the Third Age •AGE, the European Older People's Platform Age Action Ireland Age & Opportunity, Ireland Ageing and Ethnicity Web Alzheimer Europe Berlin Aging Study (BASE) Deutsches Zentrum für Alternsforschung Deutsches Zentrum ür Altersfragen The ESA Research Network on Ageing in Europe The European Commission, Ageing Policy EURAG, European Federation of the Elderly TNO Centre for Ageing Research, Leiden, Netherlands Gerontoogy in the Netherlands International Federation of Associations of the Elderly (FIAPA) MediaAge Monitoing the Regional Implementation Strategy Older Women's Network, Europe Portal Mayores, Spain Reearch roup on Aging and the Life Course (FALL), Berlin SENIORWEB, Austria SENIORWEB, Netherlands The ocial erontology Group, Department of Sociology, Uppsala University, Sweden TÁRKI, Hungary Third Age uidance World Health Organisation, Geneva, Switzerland, Library Catalogue, Health topic: Aging

Middle East

- The Program on Aging, JDC-Brookdale Institute, Israel
- www.arabscientist.org
- http://www.me-jaa.com/

Asia

- HelpAge India
- Tokyo Metropolitan Institute of Gerontology, Japan

Australasia

- Alzheimer's Association New South Wales
- Alzheimer's Australia
- Council on the Ageing
- National Ageing Research Institute, Melbourne
- Department for Communities, Western Australia
- Office for Senior Citizens, New Zealand
- The Older People and Life project, University of Sydney

North America

- Administration on Aging (USA)   Alzheimer's Association, Chicago, Illinois
- Alzheimer's Disease Research (American Health Assistance Foundation)
- AARP (formerly American Association of Retired Persons), ..
- Ageline   The Canadian Centre for Elder Law Studies (CCELS)
- Cyberseniors   Department of Elder Affairs, Florida
- ElderCare Web, Aging, Death and Dying
- Fifty Plus Net (Canadian Association of Retired Persons)
- The University of Georgia Gerontology Center
- Gerontology Research Centre, Simon Fraser University, Vancouver, Canada
- GeroWeb, Wayne State University, Institute of Gerontology, Detroit, Michigan
- Global Action on Aging   Health and Age   Health Web: Geriatrics & Gerontology
- Institute for Human Development, Life Course and Aging, University of Toronto, Canada
- International Association of Gerontology, Canada
- International Association of Homes and Services for the Ageing
- International Federation on Ageing   International Network for the Prevention of Elder Abuse
- Leadership Council of Aging Organisations
- The National Archive of Computerized Data on Aging
- National Aging Information Center, Washington DC
- National Library of Medicine , Medline
- Population Aging Research Center, University of Pennsylvania

- Portals Aging Seniornet Seniors Computer Information Project, Manitoba, Canada

American Association of Retired Persons (AARP)
601 E St., NW
Washington, DC 20049
202/434-2277
American Society on Aging (ASA)
833 Market St., Suite 511
San Francisco, CA 94103
415/974-9600
National Association of Area Agencies on Aging (NAAAA)
1112 16th St., NW, Suite 100
Washington, DC 20036
202/296-8130
National Association of State Units on Aging (NASUA)
1225 I St., NW, Suite 725
Washington, DC 20005
202/898-2578
National Institute on Aging (NIA)
Public Information Office
9000 Rockville Pike
Bethesda, MD 20892
301/496-1752
US Administration on Aging (AoA)
330 Independence Ave., SW
Washington, DC 20201
202/619-0441
US Bureau of the Census
Age and Sex Statistics Branch
Population Division
Washington, DC 20233
301/457-2378

21. Endorsements

What people are saying about "EnjoyVity-Your Full Spectrum of Life":

"I would definitely recommend it."

"This is a lucid and well researched book. Given that all readers are concerned about their health and their aging, each of you will gain insight into his or hers own health, and learn about sound balanced solutions."

~ Yves Gillard M.D., Aix-en Provence, France.

"It really contains so much useful information."

"I found the sections on detox-cleaning, aging and healthy drinking especially helpful. I really found the tips and suggestions very inspiring, positive, and motivating. Yes, it really contains so much useful information."

~David Spears, Washington, USA.

"A blue print of anti-aging."

"In his book, the author draws upon a number of key issues that play a role in both getting and staying healthy. His is an easy to read discourse on healthy living with useful tips along the way. The take home message is that healthy living doesn't have to be difficult. Much of the advice presented is the blue print of anti-ageing and naturopathic clinics, including mine."

~Han van de Braak BSc LicAc MCSP MBAcC, Chartered Physiotherapist, Registered Acupuncturist, Naturopath, London, UK.

"Book of books."

"In a simple and clear manner all facets of the HUMAN comes under the loupe. The 4-dimensional HUMAN is mapped. The HUMAN as a body, as ghost-power, as emotional motivator and as spiritual being. In short 'EnjoyVity' is for me the book of books.

~ *André De Zutter,* ear- nose- throat –allergologue , chartered **M.D., Acupuncturist, Homeopath, Neural-, Ozon-, Meso-, Orthomolecular- Enzyme-** and Oligo therapist, *Antwerp, Belgium.*

22. The "EnjoyVity" spirit brings You and many others HOPE

We are passionate about helping you "take control of your health" and sharing this vital information with you, which can radically change your health for the better.

"**EnjoyVity**" it was me yesterday, it can be or is You today and it will be our team tomorrow.

> "EnjoyVity" **stands or will stand for a**
> **Life philosophy**
> **Behavior**
> **Search for Happiness**
> **Team spirit**
> **Beautiful feeling**
> **Dream in the make**
> **Way out**
> **Way in**
> **Challenge**
> **Universal approach**
> **Shape your future**
> **Pure way to success**
> **Your full Spectrum of Life**
> ....

Longevity= long life ~ life expectancy (especially when it concerns someone or something lasting longer than expected)

"**EnjoyVity**" = enjoy life ~life in happiness ~ have a good time in life (en-joy= en joie)

"**EnjoyVitalic**" = *life sensualist, enjoying vital lifestyle and good health into his or her very old age*

Fill in your feeling, meaning and ideas about "**EnjoyVity**" and send us those

www.enjoyvity.com/ebook/

Let us learn to hope again

The unbelievable story of mankind on our planet earth in this endless Universe

Optimism

Laugh
   Joke inspiring ones and quotes on website www.enjoyvity.com/ebook/

Take hope from ...
   Read hopeful short-stories of "**Enjoy Vitalic**" team members on our website at www.enjoyvity.com

Give hope to your fellow ...
   Send in your story on how the "**Enjoy Vity**®" spirit made it happen
   - For you ...

   - For those 3 billion and growing in 3th and 4th world .....

Why to support NGO's helping children (and especially adoption)?
   Brain starts working from month 6 in mother's womb. No mother gives child for adoption without having serious life problems themselves before, during and after their pregnancy. Child starts with wrong program in its life. Who knows when and how to re-program his own not to speak of a child's brain. Let us support/sponsor research in relation with children diseases, adoption problems, mothers, ...

Sponsor: 'hungerandthirst.net' or 'savethechildren.org' or 'medecinsdumonde.org/gb/nos_missions/etranger/adoption' or 'concern.net' or 'feedthechildren.org' or 'supportunicef.org' or 'bbc.co.uk/pudsey/donate/' or of course the one of your choice.

And engage in **'child-aid'** projects yourself. **They all thank you!**

We will post regularly updates on positive findings about many of the hot subjects.
As there are Obesitas, Stress, Alzheimer, ...

Go to 'Enjoyvity.com/secrets' or

Subscribe on the website to our FREE *EnjoyVity* Newsletter 'enjoyvity.com'

Protection of private: Enjoyvity does not rent, sell or share your Personal Information with third parties except to provide products or services that you have requested, with your permission.

23. Content

	Foreword	page 5
1.	Introduction	page 7
2.	Live and make *your* life	page 11
3.	Know how to think	page 19
4.	Keep it physical	page 25
5.	Know how and what to eat	page 35
6.	Know how to drink	page 81
7.	Know how to look	page 99
8.	Know how to clean-up	page 107
9.	Have clear and clean thoughts	page 131
10.	Know how to speak	page 141
11.	Follow their 100+ example	page 147
12.	Enjoy a healthy partner, family and everlasting sex live	page 161
13.	Auto-diagnose and Self-treat	page 169
14.	Live YOUR dreams	page 175
15.	Create your paradise	page 191
16.	MY golden age, up to and over 100	page 195
17.	The 7 basic "**Enjoy** Vity" rules	page 201
18.	My Personal **Full Spectrum of life**	page 203
19.	Inspiring quotes and readings	page 207
20.	Acknowledgements and accountability	page 211
21.	Endorsements	page 215
22.	The "**Enjoy** Vity" spirit brings You and many others HOPE	page 217
23.	Content	page 221
24.	Postscript	page 223
25.	Tables	page 225
26.	Index	page 239

24. Postscript

Dear reader, the journey did not come to an end we will continue to inform you by newsletter sign up NOW http://www.enjoyvity.com/ebook/

If you found the **Enjoy**Vity approach valuable you may want to help to spread the positive spirit to friends, colleagues, ... you can do this by sending the Free introduction 'enjoyvity.com/buzz.pdf' or the link to our website 'enjoyvity.com'.

You can download and add our colorful banner to your email signature ....
Or why not send the book to your friend, colleague, ... as a gift?

Order at an extra discount rate your Gift certificate ... Or type: "deals-on-enjoyvity" in "your promotion code" module of the website to have the eBook at a rebate price!

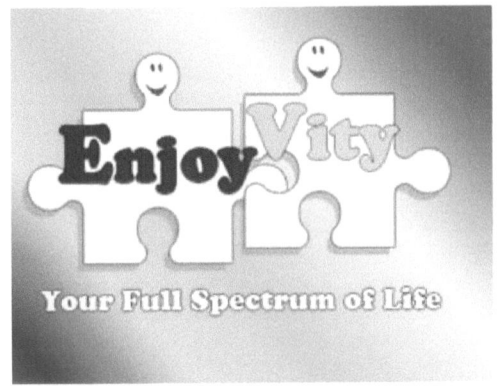

Put the number in the download area at www.enjoyvity.com/ebook

This is what your friends will receive with your Gift certificate

Your Free Wallpapers download at 'enjoyvity.com/ebook/goodies'

EnjoyVity Harmony

This book is intended to be distributed, as part of the "**Enjoy**Vity" approach. If you wish to share this document with someone, please direct them to www.enjoyvity.com and ask them to sign up for a FREE introduction.

25. Tables

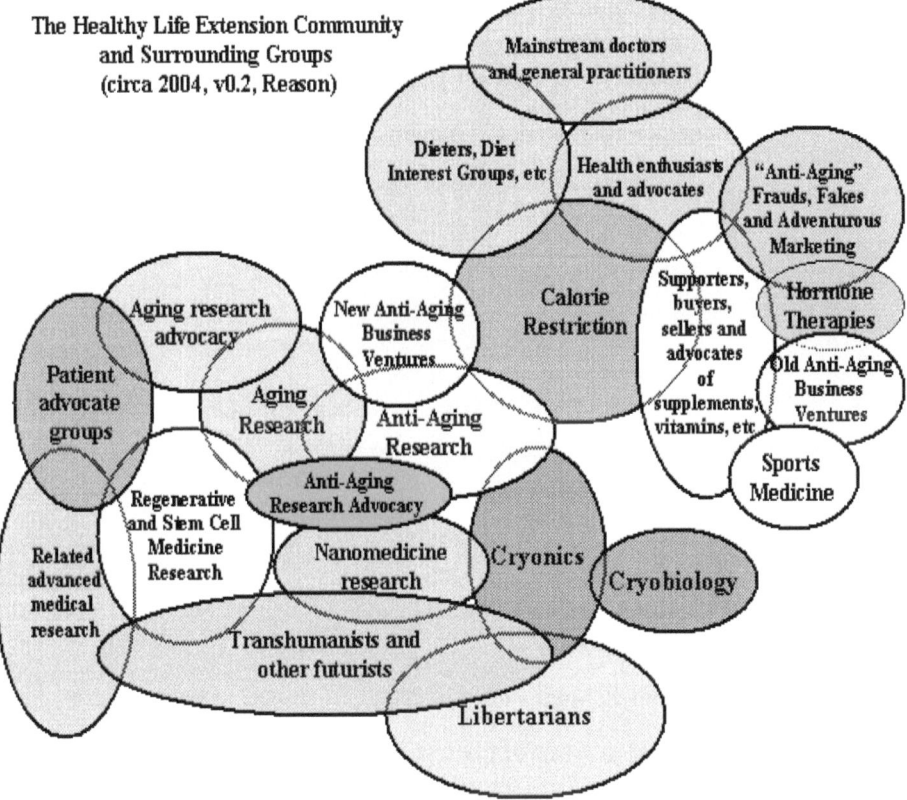

Overlapping balloons in the community visualization indicate areas of common interest and communities that share a sizeable number of members. It is interesting to note that, up until comparatively recently, parts of the community were very isolated from one another. The cryonics, calorie restriction, supplement advocates, and anti-aging research and advocacy communities have grown closer only since the advent of the Internet. This modern ease of communication opens up enormous opportunities for growth in the healthy life extension community, since everyone has wider access to the "feeder groups" (libertarians, transhumanists, extropians, dieters, health enthusiasts, and so forth) that are closely associated with parts of the wider community.

USA-Statistics

There are 20.8 million children and adults in the United States, or 7% of the population, who have diabetes. While an estimated 14.6 million have been diagnosed, unfortunately, 6.2 million people (or nearly one-third) are unaware that they have the disease.

America's Five Fastest-Growing Health Concerns

	2001	1999
Obesity*	61.0%	56.4%
Diabetes	18.3%	12.0%
Depression	19.1%	14.8%
Impotence	9.2%	7.4%
Aging Related Problems	22.5%	19.2%

* In 1980, the national average of obese adults was 15 percent. In 1991 it was already 27%.

USA Obesity Rates Reach Epidemic Proportions

- 58 Million Overweight; 40 Million Obese; 3 Million morbidly Obese
- Eight out of 10 over 25's Overweight
- 78% of American's not meeting basic activity level recommendations
- 25% completely Sedentary
- 76% increase in Type II diabetes in adults 30-40 yrs old since 1990

Obesity-Related Diseases

- 80% of type II diabetes related to obesity
- 70% of Cardiovascular disease related to obesity
- 42% breast and colon cancer diagnosed among obese individuals
- 30% of gall bladder surgery related to obesity
- 26% of obese people having high blood pressure

Obesity Related Disease Costs Overwhelm HealthCare System

- Type II Diabetes ($63.14 Billion)
- Osteoporosis ($17.2 Billion)
- Hypertension ($3.23 Billion)
- Heart Disease ($6.99 Billion)
- Post-menopausal breast cancer ($2.32 Billion)
- Colon Cancer ($2.78 Billion)
- Endometrial Cancer ($790 Million)

Cost of Lost Productivity

- Workdays lost: $39.3 Million
- Physician office visits: $62.7 Million
- Restricted Activity days: $29.9 Million
- Bed-Related days: $89.5 Million

Childhood Obesity Running Out of Control

- 4% overweight 1982 | 16% overweight 1994
- 25% of all white children overweight 2001
- 33% African American and Hispanic children overweight 2001
- Hospital costs associated with childhood obesity rising from $35 Million (1979) to $127 Million (1999)
- New study suggests one in four overweight children is already showing early signs of type II diabetes (impaired glucose intolerance)
- 60% already have one risk factor for heart disease

Surge in Childhood Diabetes

- Between 8% - 45% of newly diagnosed cases of childhood diabetes are type II, associated with obesity.
- Whereas 4% of Childhood diabetes was type II in 1990, that number has risen to approximately 20%
- Depending on the age group (Type II most frequent 10-19 group) and the racial/ethnic mix of group stated
- Of Children diagnosed with Type II diabetes, 85% are obese

This research information was prepared by independent authors. It has been reproduced in its entirety or as a collection of information gathered from multiple resources and research data. 'EnjoyVity' is not liable for any inaccuracies found in any third party written articles or research. References: National Institute of Diabetes & Digestive & Kidney Diseases (NIDDK) and My.WebMD.com website.

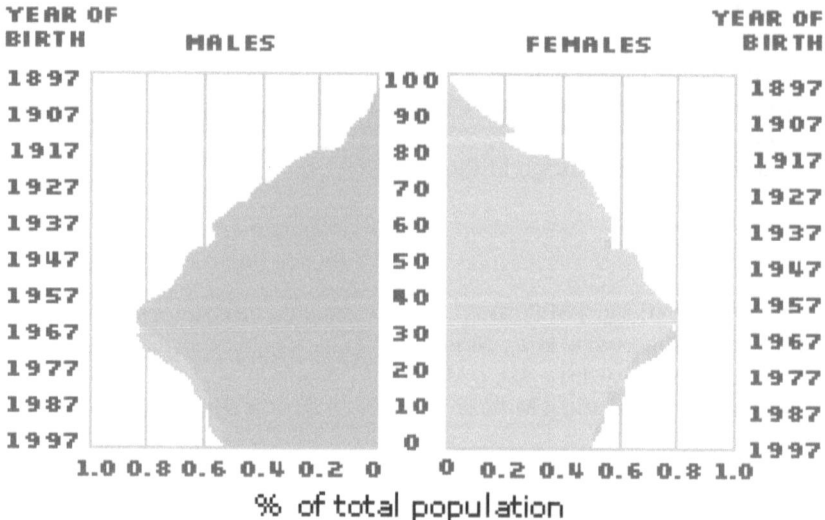

Worldwide the population 60 and over is growing faster than any other group. The 60+ population, at 605 million in 2009 will double by 2025 and reach 2 billion by 2050.

An estimated 46-million Americans have no health insurance and more than 108-million people in the US are without dental insurance. Nearly one-quarter of the uninsured reported changing their way of life significantly in order to pay medical bills. Almost half of the two-million Americans who file for bankruptcy do so because of medical expenses.

Population Pyramid Summary for United States / *Source: U.S. Census Bureau*

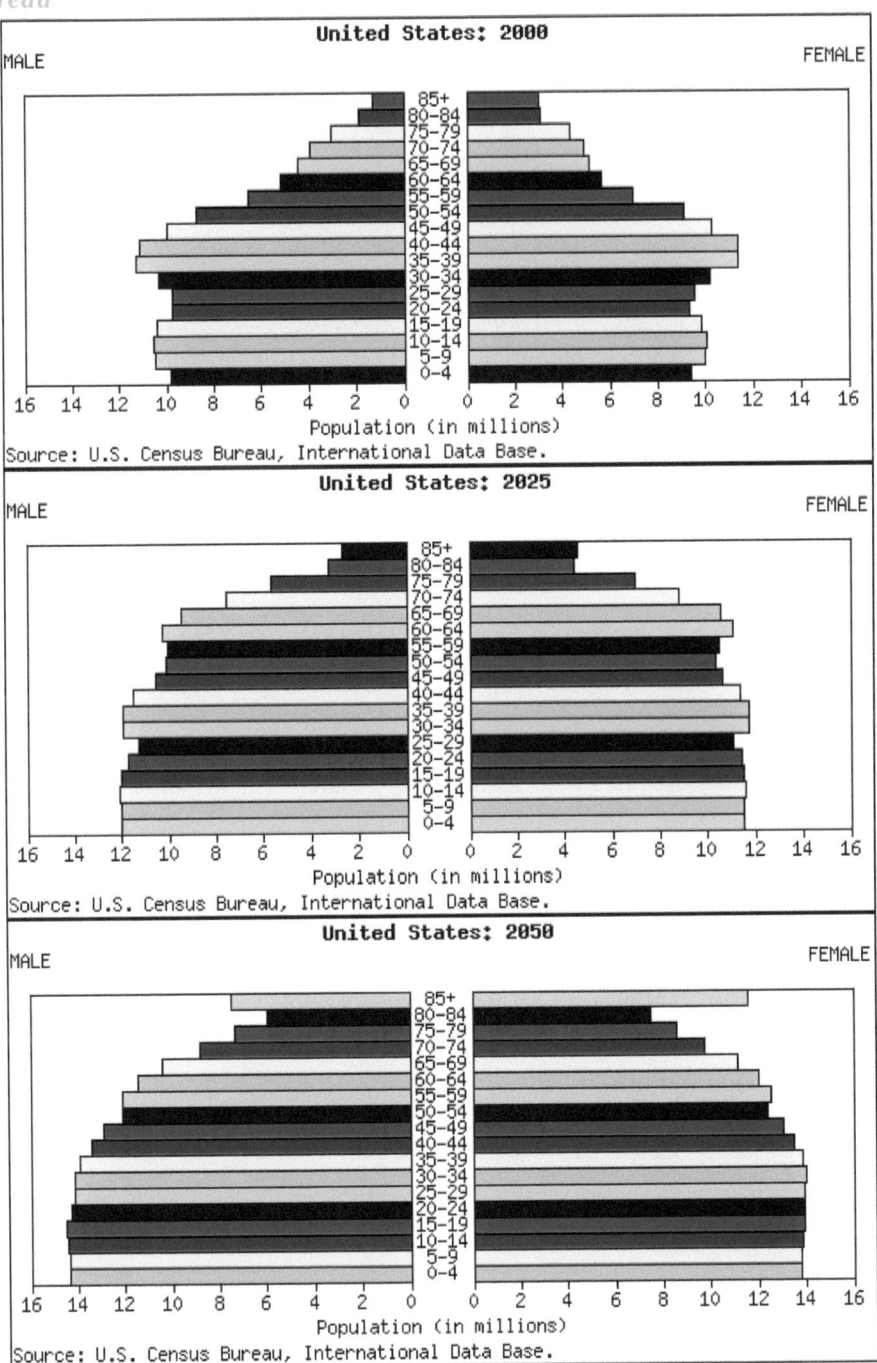

How do the generations compare?

	18 - 34 yr olds	35 - 53 yr olds	55 and older
smoke more than a half a pack of cigarettes a day	17%	21%	14%
have a chronic disease or condition requiring regular care	8%	20%	49%
use vitamins or supplements or try to eat mostly organic foods	42%	51%	60%
almost always read labels to find out about content of food	59%	63%	64%
have a stressful job or frequently feel a great deal of stress	47%	57%	20%
restrict the amount of red meat they eat	36%	49%	51%
have checked their blood pressure or cholesterol in the past year	71%	78%	94%
could easily run or jog a mile	70%	46%	22%
have a family doctor	78%	78%	91%
drink three or more cups of coffee a day	15%	32%	30%
regularly do yoga meditation or other stress reducing exercises	24%	25%	20%
drink an alcoholic beverage almost every day	9%	11%	14%

From the Wall Street Journal, June 28, 1996

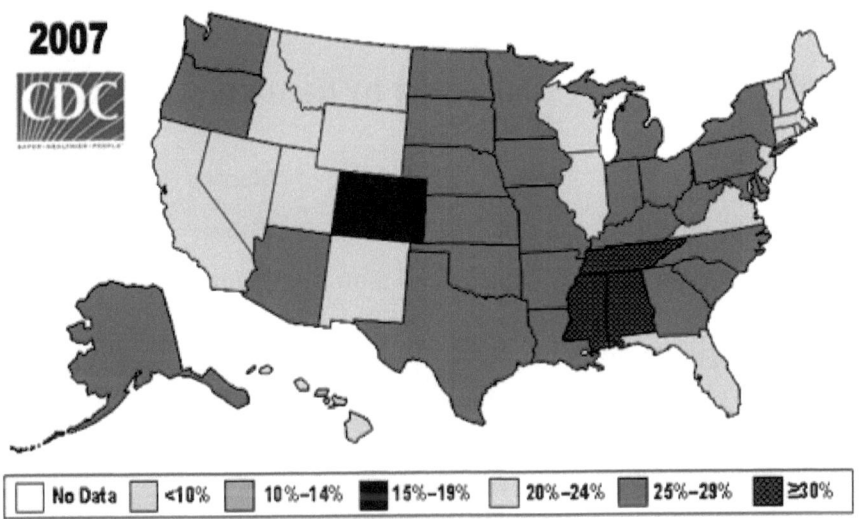

Percent of Obese (BMI ≥ 30) in U.S. Adults ~CDC 2008

Hours spent per day on activities*

ACTIVITY	MEN	WOMEN
Sleep	8:29	8:39
Housework	1:10	1:48
Food prep / cleanup	0:44	1:12
Caring for household children	1:31	2:08
Caring for household members	1:39	2:19
Work	7:59	7:02
Attending class	5:26	4:51
Homework / research	2:32	2:28
Religion / spiritual activities	1:50	1:42
Volunteering	2:23	2:01
Watching TV	3:26	3:07
Sports / exercise	2:01	1:20

*by respondents reporting participation in that activity.   SOURCE: US DEPARTMENT OF LABOR

(These figures are averages of all respondents' answers. The graph below reflects only the time of people who reported taking part in those activities.)

ACTIVITY	TIME SPENT BY GENDER, MARITAL STATUS			
	Men	Women	Married	Single
Phone calls, mail, e-mail	7 min.	14 min.	8 min.	14 min.
Caring for non-household members	13 min.	15 min.	13 min.	14 min.
Religious, civic duties	16 min.	21 min.	20 min.	17 min.
Caring for family	20 min.	43 min.	45 min.	17 min.
Educational activities	28 min.	26 min.	7 min.	51 min.
Buying goods, services	38 min.	58 min.	53 min.	42 min.
Eating, drinking	1 hr. 18 min.	1 hr. 11 min.	1 hr. 24 min.	1 hr. 8 min.
Household activities	1 hr. 20 min.	2 hr. 16 min.	2 hr. 8 min.	1 hr. 26 min.
Work-related	4 hr. 26 min.	3 hr.	4 hr. 1 min.	3 hr. 18 min.
Watching TV	3 hr. 28 min.	2 hr. 41 min.	2 hr. 24 min.	2 hr. 47 min.
Personal care, sleep	9 hr. 13 min.	9 hr. 37 min.	9 hr. 8 min.	9 hr. 46 min.

Sources:

Having More Leisure Time —Federal Reserve Bank of Boston, "Measuring Trends in Leisure: The Allocation of Time over Five Decades" *Numbers of People Doing Activities* —Statistical abstract of the United States, 2004

Volume (Dry)

American Standard	Metric
1/8 teaspoon	.5 ml
1/4 teaspoon	1 ml
1/2 teaspoon	2 ml
3/4 teaspoon	4 ml
1 teaspoon	5 ml
1 tablespoon	15 ml
1/4 cup	59 ml
1/3 cup	79 ml
1/2 cup	118 ml
2/3 cup	158 ml
3/4 cup	177 ml
1 cup	225 ml
2 cups or 1 pint	450 ml
3 cups	675 ml
4 cups or 1 quart	1 liter
1/2 gallon	2 liters
1 gallon	4 liters

Volume (Liquid)

American Standard (Cups & Quarts)	American Standard (Ounces)	Metric (Milliliters & Liters)
2 tbsp	1 fl. oz.	30 ml
1/4 cup	2 fl. oz.	60 ml
1/2 cup	4 fl. oz.	125 ml
1 cup	8 fl. oz.	250 ml
1 1/2 cups	12 fl. oz.	375 ml
2 cups or 1 pint	16 fl. oz.	500 ml
4 cups or 1 quart	32 fl. oz.	1000 ml or 1 liter
1 gallon	128 fl. oz.	4 liters

Oven Temperatures

American Standard	Metric
250° F	130° C
300° F	150° C
350° F	180° C
400° F	200° C
450° F	230° C

Weight (Mass)

American Standard (Ounces)	Metric (Grams)
1/2 ounce	15 grams
1 ounce	30 grams
3 ounces	85 grams
3.75 ounces	100 grams
4 ounces	115 grams
8 ounces	225 grams
12 ounces	340 grams
16 ounces or 1 pound	450 grams

Dry Measure Equivalents

3 teaspoons	1 tablespoon	1/2 ounce	14.3 grams
2 tablespoons	1/8 cup	1 ounce	28.3 grams
4 tablespoons	1/4 cup	2 ounces	56.7 grams
5 1/3 tablespoons	1/3 cup	2.6 ounces	75.6 grams
8 tablespoons	1/2 cup	4 ounces	113.4 grams
12 tablespoons	3/4 cup	6 ounces	.375 pound
32 tablespoons	2 cups	16 ounces	1 pound

British and American Variances

Term	Abbreviation	Nationality	Dry or liquid	Metric equivalent	Equivalent in context
cup	c., C.		usually liquid	237 milliliters	16 tablespoons or 8 ounces
ounce	fl oz, fl. oz.	American	liquid only	29.57 milliliters	
		British	either	28.41 milliliters	
gallon	gal.	American	liquid only	3.785 liters	4 quarts
		British	either	4.546 liters	4 quarts
inch	in, in.			2.54 centimeters	
ounce	oz, oz.	American	dry	28.35 grams	1/16 pound
			liquid	see OUNCE	see OUNCE
pint	p., pt.	American	liquid	0.473 liter	1/8 gallon or 16 ounces
			dry	0.551 liter	1/2 quart
		British	either	0.568 liter	
pound	lb.		dry	453.592 grams	16 ounces
quart	q., qt, qt.	American	liquid	0.946 liter	1/4 gallon or 32 ounces
			dry	1.101 liters	2 pints
		British	either	1.136 liters	
teaspoon	t., tsp., tsp		either	about 5 milliliters	1/3 tablespoon
tablespoon	T., tbs., tbsp.		Either	about 15 milliliters	3 teaspoons or 1/2 ounce

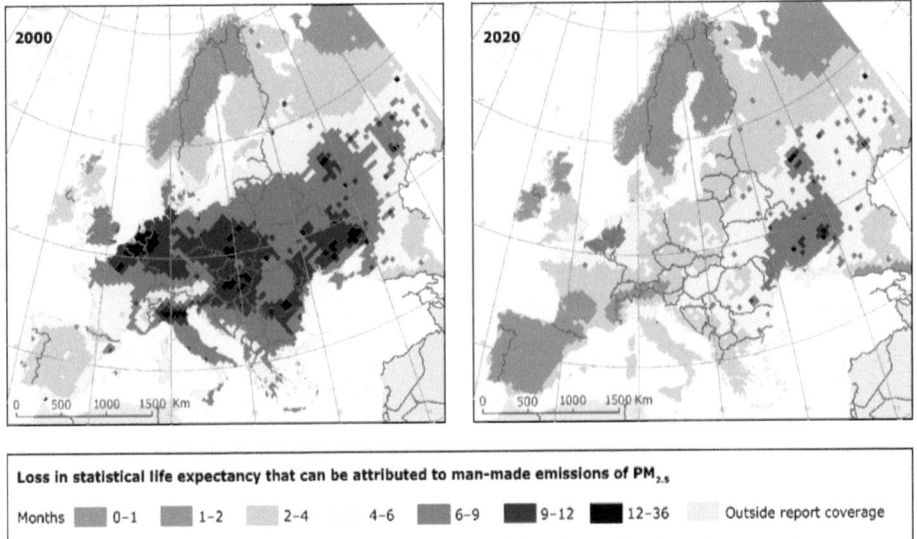

European Environment Agency *from* A further emission control scenario for the Clean Air For Europe (CAFE) program.

BioElectroniqueVincent/Medical

Evaluation Sheet

Firma Med-Tronik GmbH
Forschung & Entwicklung
Daimlerstr. 2
D-77948 Friesenheim
07821/6333-0

Date: 30.07.98

Surname:	Barta			Date of measurement:	26.02.98
First name:	Josef			Age:	57 Years
Birth date:	16.04.41				

Measurement	pH	rH2	R	Evaluation	PHP	118.00
Blood	7.41	23.30	217		RHP	63.75
Saliva	7.40	26.90	242		RP	5.98
Urine I	5.79	22.50	105	Liquids	Quantity at	88 kg
Urine II	5.65	21.50	87		Blood 3.94 Lt	298 µW 1174 x Vol
Urine III					Saliva 1.01 Lt	544 µW 501 x Vol
					Urine 1.10 Lt	1076 µW 1184 x Vol
				Factor C		0.72
				Defense factor:		4.24 Vi
Normal:	pH	rH2	R	Active potential:		2.29 PA
Blood	7.30	22	210	Integral value:		5.7 FG
Saliva	6.50	22	190	IW s rated value		36.63 IW%
Urine	5.80	24	30			

Defense situation

Thrombosis Risk

Relative assessment

Blood: WITHOUT DIAGNOSIS
Saliva: ACUTE OR CHRONICAL OCCURRENCE IN THE DIGESTIVE SYSTEM
DEFICIENCY OF ENZYMES
METALS IN THE ORAL CAVITY? BLOCKAGE OF THE PANCREAS AREA? DENTAL FOCUS?
MASSIVE LYMPHATIC STRESS
ALKALOSIS OF SALIVA
Urine: LATENT MESENCHYMAL ACIDOSIS
RESTRICTED FUNCTION OF THE KIDNEYS

The diagnosis obtained by using the procedures of BEV may not always coincide with a clinical manifestation of the indicated illness (subjective complaints and clinical objectifying diagnosis). However the BEV diagnosis does in any case indicate tendency processes with respect to the indicated illness.

USDA data on foods with high levels of antioxidant phytochemicals

Food	Serving size	Antioxidant capacity per serving size
Cinnamon, ground	100 grams	267,536
Aronia black chokeberry (*Aronia melanocarpa*)	100 grams	16062
Small Red Bean	½ cup dried beans	13727
Wild blueberry	1 cup	13427
Red kidney bean *	½ cup dried beans	13259
Pinto bean	½ cup	11864
Blueberry	1 cup (cultivated berries)	9019
Cranberry	1 cup (whole berries)	8983
Artichoke hearts	1 cup, cooked	7904
Blackberry	1 cup (cultivated berries)	7701
Prune	½ cup	7291
Raspberry	1 cup	6058
Strawberry	1 cup	5938
Red Delicious apple	1 apple	5900
Granny Smith apple	1 apple	5381

Pecan	1 oz	5095
Sweet cherry	1 cup	4873
Black plum	1 plum	4844
Russet potato	1, cooked	4649
Black bean	½ cup dried beans	4181
Plum	1 plum	4118
Gala apple	1 apple	3903

26. INDEX

A

acid deposits · 43
Acupressure
  shiatsu · 108
additive · 28
AGEs · 65
Air
  therapy · 77
Alan L.Watson · 25
Alcohol
  BAC · 60
Alkaemia · 50
alkaline foods · 49
Aloe supplement · 65
Alzheimer
  prevention · 89
Alzheimer Association · 3
Amalgam · 89
American Journal of Physical
  Anthropology · 14
Anti-Aging · 65
Antioxidants · 47
apiary
  collectif · 120
Aristoteles · 9
Avocados · 40
Ayurveda · 108
  tongue diagnosis · 74

B

bedroom · 117
berries · 41
Bioelectronic · 61
biological clock · 115
Biorhythm · 38
birch
  detox juice · 75
birch juice · 75
Blue Zone · 97
BMI · 32
BMR · 34
body language · 90
Boomers · 3
brain
  waves · 87
Breath · 110
breathing
  diaphragm · 79
Buckwheat · 41

C

Cacao
  catechins · 59
Calorie restriction · 38
cells
  trillion · 69
centenarian
  Azerbeidjan, Kreta · 98
centennials

Hunza · 95
champagne
  as brain protection · 61
chew
  chewing · 24
Chew · 23
  30 times · 23
Choi and Yu
  iron overdose · 58
Chopra Deepak · 132
CLA · 29
Claude Bernard
  terrain · 61
cleaning
  blood · 73
  colon · 73
  liver · 72, 73
  spring · 72
  Spring · 72
coaching · 68
Cobra · 19
Cod liver oil · 31
COKE
  exercises · 111
color
  personal · 67
Color
  therapy · 77
Confucius · 13
Conspiracy of the Rich
  R.Kiyosaki · 85
cosmic energy · 103
cosmos
  macro · 81
Cultured vegetables · 40

D

Dale Carnegie · 12
David Paterson · 28
David Wolfe · 22
de-stress · 5
DESTRESS · 116
detox
  general · 74
Detox
  algae · 74
  clay · 74
detoxification · 72
dew walk · 20
diabetes · 25
diarrhea · 75
Doctor Jeanne Rousseau · 75
dream
  REM · 118
Dream
  lucid · 118
  recall · 118
drinking
  AAA · 62

E

electrosmog
  NY · 86
Emotional
  EFT · 88
EnjoyVity®
  rules · 128
enzymes · 23
Eons
  calculator · 126
epidemical' · 23
Extinction · 119

F

F.D.Roosevelt · 13
Family · 105
Fast Reading

time gain · 92
Fasting · 74
Feedbag · 46
Feng Shui · 67
Fermented · 39
ferments · 74
ferments of life · 102
    Lesik · 74
Fernanda Amicarelli
    ELF-MF · 85
Fibers · 40
Flax Seed · 42
Fluor · 54
Food Pyramid · 25
Frank Sacks · 23
FREE
    ebook · 106
free electrons · 55
French Paradox
    resveratrol · 60

G

galaxy
    M-51 · 81
    sagittarius dwarf · 70
Garladior · 44
Garlic · 42
Generation-X · 3
Generation-Y · 3
George Bernard Shaw · 7, 16, 108
George Chaplin · 14
Gift certificate · 143
Ginger · 43
Guru · 15

H

HappyBook · 88
Harvard School · 23, 25

Helen Keller · 8
Hirotada Ototake · 12
holistic · 14, 23
Homeopathics · 110
homo sapiens · 23
Honeybees · 119
Hormonal · 109
Horseradish · 41
Human Growth Hormones · 38
hunter-gatherer · 23

I

Infrared
    cabin · 78
intuition · 112
inulin' · 42
ioniser
    air · 87

J

J.Yves Verheyen · 10
James C. Riley · 124
James Fowler, UC San Diego · 28
Joan Welsh · 16

K

Karl Loren · 46
Kefir · 40
Kegel
    PC exercise · 107
Keizo Miura
    routine · 101
kinesiology
    applied · 109
Kinesiology
    braingym · 88
Kneipp

body and mind balance · 71
Kuhne
   ice pack · 71

L

L.C.Vincent
   bioelectronic · 61
Lauri Quinn Loewenberg · 118
Lesik™ · 74
Lévi-Strauss · 120
life expectancy
   history · 124
Life expectancy
   record · 125
loneliness · 91
longevity · 98
Louis Pasteur · 12
love
   yourself · 123

M

Made in Africa · 14
magic pill · 39
Mark Twain · 6
Maya Angelou
   dare · 83
Meditate · 85
Mediterranean diet · 46
Mesenchyme · 49
MET · 36
metabolism · 36
metabolism boosters · 37
Michael Anthony
   HappyBook · 88
Mike Dooley
   TuT · 84
Minerals
   and aging · 96

miracle diet · 23
MODERATION · 32
muscles not fat · 20
Music
   therapy · 78

N

network
   build · 92
networking · 106
Nina Jablonski · 14
Nutrigenetics · 97

O

obesity · 26, 28
Okinawans · 47
omega 6 · 29
ORAC · 41
ORP
   redox · 82
Orthomolecular
   anti-aging · 126
orthorexia · 37
overweight · 33

P

Paradise · 122
partner
   polygyny · 104
Patrick Flanagan
   crystal energy · 96
pH · 49
philosophical · 113
phones
   mobile · 83
pilates · 16
Pomegranate · 39

PRAL · 50
probiotics · 39
processed · 28
protein · 26
Psychognomy
   Paul Bouts · 99

Q

Qigong · 17

R

Rachel Carson · 29
REAL CHANGE · 15
Regulator
   biological · 75
   weight · 75
Rene Quinton
   Plasma · 96
Repetition · 16
Reverse List · 48
rH2 · 50
Rhonda Byrne
   The secret · 104
Richard Cutler · 47
Robert Kiyosaki · 7
Rooibos · 58

S

Sainkho Namtchylak · 13
Sauna
   banya · 78
Scientific American
   aging · 94
Seaweed · 43
Sherry Tenpenny
   no to vaccines · 61
Shri Mataji · 13

Sixth Great Extinction · 119
Sleep
   amount · 114
   sleep apnea · 116
Slow Food · 46
Snoring
   apnea · 116
SOT-point · 109
Soybean · 48
speak
   confident · 92
spirit · 139
Spirit · 13
Sri Swami Buaji Maharaj
   +118 · 98
Steambath · 78
stool · 72
   slow · 72
storyofstuff · 7
stress
   oxidative · 82
Stress
   SOT · 109
stretching · 16
supplements · 38

T

Tai-Chi · 16, 17
Tea
   black · 57
   green · 57
   Oolong · 57
   white · 57
terrain
   emotional · 129
   physical · 129
therapy
   aroma · 110
   reflex · 108

Thomas Perls
   ageing · 94
Thorax · 19
top 10 of cities · 10
tut.com · 8

V

vaccination · 61
vegetable
   juices · 59
Viagra
   natural & free · 106
Vilcabamba · 97
Vincent · 61

W

Walter Breuning
   +102 · 100
Walter C. Willett · 25
Walter D. Wintle · 84
Warburg · 61
water
   alkaline · 56
   functions · 54
   ionized · 55
   needs · 53
   which · 54
weight loss · 25
Weight training · 20
Weston A. Price
   tribal diets · 98
WHO · 27
WiFi
   mobile · 86
Winston Churchill · 84

Y

yawning · 5, 117
yoga · 113
   face · 117

Z

Zero-Neck-Roll · 18

"*C.O.K.E.*" times 8!

Make "*C.O.K.E*" your favorites; repetition is key for success, do at least 4 per day and rotate through them on a regular basis. Become an "**Enjoy**Vity" master.

 1. Zero Neck Roll

 2. Smile

 3. Kuhne's (ice packing)

 4. Kegel's (pubis squeeze)

 5. SOT Point

 6. Deep Breath

 7. Einstein's (lion pause)

 8. Yawn   *tear out and use at your convenience*   © enjoyvity.com

www.ingramcontent.com/pod-product-compliance
Ingram Content Group UK Ltd.
Pitfield, Milton Keynes, MK11 3LW, UK
UKHW041257180426
11947UKWH00008B/538